_**Healing
Mind,
Body,
Spirit**_

Also by M. J. Abadie

Your Psychic Potential

Child Signs

Love Planets
(with Claudia Bader)

Finding Love
(with Sally Jessy Raphael)

Healing Mind, Body, Spirit

M. J. Abadie

Adams Media Corporation
Holbrook, Massachusetts

Copyright © 1997 by M. J. Abadie. All rights reserved.
This book, or parts thereof, may not be reproduced in any form
without permission from the publisher; exceptions are made
for brief excerpts used in published reviews.

Published by
Adams Media Corporation
260 Center Street, Holbrook, MA 02343

ISBN: 1-55850-716-7
Printed in the United States of America.

First Edition
J I H G F E D C B A

Library of Congress Cataloging-in-Publication Data
Abadie, M. J. (Marie-Jeanne)
Healing mind, body, spirit / M. J. Abadie.—1st ed.
p. cm.
Includes bibliographical references.
ISBN 1-55850-716-7
1. Astrology and health. 2. Healing—Miscellanea. 3. Alternative healing.
4. Mind and body. I. Title.
BF1729.H9A23   1997
615.8'56—dc21   97-6830
CIP

This publication is designed to provide accurate and authoritative information with regard to the subject matter covered. It is sold with the understanding that the publisher is not engaged in rendering legal, accounting, or other professional advice. If legal advice or other expert assistance is required, the services of a competent professional person should be sought.
— From a *Declaration of Principles* jointly adopted by a Committee of the American Bar Association and a Committee of Publishers and Associations

Grateful acknowledgment is made to North Atlantic Books for permission to reprint excerpts from *The Alchemy of Healing: Psyche & Soma* by Edward C. Whitmont © 1992.

Cover photo by Tim Flach/©Tony Stone Images

This book is available at quantity discounts for bulk purchases.
For information, call 1-800-872-5627 (in Massachusetts, 617-767-8100).

Visit our home page at http://www.adamsmedia.com

To
Blanche Meyerson
Friend ∾ Healer ∾ Inspiration
and
In memoriam
Robert Adrian Brouwer
of the Netherlands
1933–1996

contents

Acknowledgments / ix

Foreword
  My Search for Healing / xi

Introduction
  The Inner Dynamics of Healing / xxiii

PART ONE: PSYCHE AND SOMA

Chapter One
  The Mind-Body-Spirit Connection / 3

Chapter Two
  The Roots of Illness / 15

PART TWO: TRANSFORMATIONS OF HEALING

Chapter Three
  Healing: An Alchemical Process / 31

Chapter Four
  The Healing Journey / 43

Chapter Five
  Advice to the Traveler / 57

Healing Mind, Body, Spirit

PART THREE: THE TRANSFORMATIVE HEALING POWERS

Chapter Six
   The Healing Body / 79

Chapter Seven
   The Healing Mind / 105

Chapter Eight
   The Healing Spirit / 131

PART FOUR: THE COSMIC ORGANISM

Chapter Nine
   The Transforming Crisis / 163

Chapter Ten
   The Healing Moon / 183

Afterword
   The Serpent's Message / 215

Appendices
   Selected Bibliography / 227
   Resources / 233
   Moon Ephemeris: How to Find Your Moon Sign / 239
   Astrological and Counseling Services / 255

acknowledgments

My dear friend Blanche Meyerson is the first recipient of my gratitude, and of my admiration for her healing work, the experience of which originally inspired me to want to write a book on the subject. If the world had more healers like her, it would be a kinder, gentler place where body and soul would be treated as the unit that they intrinsically are. In hopeful anticipation of the arrival of that far-off day, I salute her pioneering efforts.

My thanks go to Charlotte Hunter for putting an important resource into my hands at just the right moment; to John Knox for insightful commentary that often illuminated my efforts; and to Mark Hasselriis whose comprehensive work on symbolism has supported my own. My researcher, Allen Erdheim, was invaluable as a bringer of information.

As one always draws on the work of those who have come before, I acknowledge the giants on whose shoulders I have stood—Joseph Campbell, Carl G. Jung, Edward C. Whitmont, and Erich Neumann in particular. Others who deserve mention are referenced in the selected Bibliography.

Healing Mind, Body, Spirit

Pam Liflander is heralded for her patience in guiding (and suffering through) the many revisions that have ensued on the journey to the printer, acting as midwife even as she was becoming a mother herself.

Mary Orser and Richard Zarro kindly gave permission for the use of the Moon Attunement, from their book *Changing Your Destiny*.

Joan Baren of Sag Harbor, N.Y., founder of the "America by Its Children" program, is thanked for her love and support over the years that we—together and separately—have pursued both art and healing, and also for the gift of some useful tapes.

The late Robert A. Brouwer is remembered for many benefits he brought to my life, one of which was the wonderful trip to Portugal mentioned herein.

And I say a heartfelt thanks for my German friend, Désirée Kahn, who facilitated my stay at the clinic in Bad Bruckenau. Without her help and hospitality I would not have had those unforgettable, truly remarkable experiences during my long stay in Germany.

It's said that one doesn't *write* a book—instead, you go out into the wilderness and wait for the Spirit of the book to speak. My experience bears this out, and no acknowledgments would be complete without mention of the support received from invisible Powers, which, though unseen, make their presence known to me every day of my life.

foreword: My Search for Healing

If I can stop one heart from
 breaking,
I shall not live in vain;
If I can ease one life the aching,
Or cool one pain,
Or help one fainting robin
Unto his nest again,
I shall not live in vain.

~ Emily Dickinson

Healing Mind, Body, Spirit

Where does a book come from? The genesis of this book lies in the circumstances of my life, which have made the quest for healing—in one form or another—a lifelong occupation.

Psychologist Carl Rogers remarked that the response from his audiences had made him realize that people are hungry to know something of the person teaching them. Since I assume the role of teacher for the time you spend reading my words, I want to give you some pertinent information about myself that will explain the impetus from which this book derives. In so doing, I reveal much that is personal. I do so not from any pleasure at self-revelation, but because I know that many of you suffer the consequences of early trauma and deprivation, and I want you to benefit from my experience.

My mother died when I was one year old. When I was two, my father agreed to my adoption by a childless couple who were friends of my mother. However, at the lawyer's office, when he was to sign the final papers and hand me over, he suddenly reneged on the arrangement in a tearfully dramatic scene that stunned the onlookers, declaring that he could never give up his little girl.

Soon thereafter, he sent me to a religious boarding school, where for seven years I received an impersonal, uncaring upbringing in the chilly, sanctity-saturated atmosphere of a Catholic convent. This institution was, paradoxically, all-female without being in the least maternal. There were no hugs and kisses, no kind and loving words, no laps in which to sit, no comforts for hurts, no sympathy for tears, no bedtime stories, no tucking-in rituals. We lived by rigid schedules for rising, chapel, classes, meals, baths, bedtime—announced by the rude clanging of a bell. Strict rules and regulations, with harsh punishment for infractions, prevailed. Often, the nuns would lock a terrified little girl overnight in a dark, unfamiliar room.

My Search for Healing

Illness was treated as a misdemeanor. A sick child was made to feel culpable—a troublemaker guilty of disrupting the routine and causing extra effort. Punishment could ensue. One time, in retaliation for throwing up after breakfast, the nuns would not allow me to attend the evening Halloween party, an event to which I had eagerly looked forward. Alone in the top-floor dormitory, from where I could hear the merriment below, I put on my dime-store gypsy costume, banged my tambourine, and imagined I lived in a gaudily painted caravan. My one joy in this bleak place was the ballet and tap-dance classes I attended weekly.

Other boarders went home on weekends and holidays. Mostly, I did not. Often I remained in residence during the nuns' summer retreat, the only child there. As the black-robed figures padded a continuous round from chapel to meals to chapel to bed to chapel in an eerie, ghostlike silence, broken only by their mumbled prayers and the clacking of the long wooden rosary beads that hung from their waists, I wandered the vacant corridors and deserted grounds unsupervised. Such circumstances drive the psyche in on itself and provide a fertile breeding ground for the imagination.

During these solitary summers, books were my sole companions. I became a voracious reader. Exhausting the children's room, I helped my unattended self to the contents of the nuns' library, which was forbidden to students. There, in a science book, I discovered the big bang theory of the origin of the universe, which flew in the face of everything I had been told about God's seven days of creation. When I questioned my teacher about this contradiction, she said that the book was wrong. However, she had already instilled in me a passionate reverence for the printed word, so I now put my trust in it rather than in the catechism indoctrination I received daily.

When I was eight, I was sent home with a case of measles, during which, as a direct result of parental negligence, I contracted polio and had my dream of becoming a dancer smashed. After months of being in bed without any physical therapy or medical attention, I made myself get up and walk. Somehow I knew that—if I was not to spend my life in a wheelchair—I had to heal myself. I limped from one leg shorter than the other and suffered excruciating pain from the muscle contractions, but there was no one to help me: I had to manage it myself. And so I did.

When I was nine, in the wake of my father's remarriage and subsequent dislocation of the family, I was taken out of the convent. At first I thought I was going to have a mother, but my stepmother's obvious enmity toward me soon dashed that yearning hope. Bounced around a succession of schools, I was friendless and isolated; and, as my father's unhappy, strife-ridden marriage deteriorated, he became increasingly alcoholic and abusive, with me as his chief target. These conditions required that I take care of myself.

As well as the after-effects of polio, I suffered chronic sore throats caused by untreated tonsillitis and severe respiratory problems that often left me gasping for breath. When my throat became painfully sore, I prayed for it to get well; when I couldn't breathe freely, I forced myself to concentrate on taking one breath at a time; when my legs locked in excruciatingly painful muscle cramps, I sat down and went limp all over until the spasms relaxed. Out of sheer necessity, unknowingly I had stumbled on basic healing principles.

During my teen years, the abuse escalated, and I prayed a lot, sometimes all night. I talked to God and got answers until, in a penetrating flash of insight, I realized that *I was talking to myself*, what today we call inner dialogue with the unconscious. As a small child, I had spent hours lying in the grass watching bugs and examining plants, totally absorbed in the minute activities of nature; when older, I tracked the moon's course across the sky and gazed at the stars far into the night—both rudimentary forms of meditation. Climbing aboard the magic carpet of my mind and imagining myself elsewhere, in different circumstances, was a form of visualization.

How far back does one look for the germinating seed of a life-view? I remember it precisely. In a flash of insight, the summer of my eleventh year, I first realized that I could *think*.

During an abusive crisis, one of many in which my father expostulated that, "If it weren't for you, your mother would be alive today," something went *click*. In a moment of dazzling perception, I understood my mind had immense powers. This totally unexpected revelation changed my life. The sudden shift into *consciousness* made me a survivor instead of a victim. Thus it was that I was able to preserve myself, my sanity, and my health.

As a result of my urgent need to understand and cope with what was going on around me, I developed a passionate interest in psychology. By thirteen, I had read through all of Freud's work and was into Kraft-Ebbing's great classic on abnormal psychology. My aim in life was to become a psychiatrist. I was fortunate that the public high school I attended had high academic standards.

At fifteen and an honor student, I graduated expecting to go directly into college, but my long-cherished dream of becoming a psychiatrist went down the drain during a ten-minute conversation with my father—the only one we ever had about my education or my future—who denied me both the funds and permission on the grounds that girls, who were expected to marry young, did not need extensive education.

An excellent command of the English language and a natural fluency with words enabled me to obtain full-time work at age sixteen. I held jobs in publishing, advertising, and broadcasting before reaching legal age, when I moved to another city. There, while barely supporting myself with a full-time job in an advertising agency, I attended a large university, but my courses were unchallenging—I felt I was not learning anything. In response to my complaints, the dean advised me to transfer to a school more commensurate with my abilities, such as Columbia University in New York.

At this time, thoroughly disillusioned with the rigid and outmoded dogma of the Catholic Church, which I openly opposed, I undertook independent study of philosophy and comparative religion, through which I encountered Joseph Campbell's *The Hero with a Thousand Faces*. This marvelous book enabled me to end my long moral struggle and finally break free of the Catholic Church. Little did I dream I'd one day work with this great man and enjoy a close relationship with him.

Then it happened that, because of my gender (in those pre-Women's Liberation days), I could make no further progress with my career. The advertising agency where I had headed an art department for two years was expanding, but my boss hired a man to run the larger department, relegating me to be his underling. This professional insult combined with my dissatisfaction with my classes made me decide to move to New York City, with the intention of attending Columbia. I got an advertising job almost immediately, but my meager salary—the only money I had—could not possibly be stretched to include the high cost of tuition. Once again, I had to shelve my ambition. Instead, with only my experience to rely on, I concentrated on a career in advertising. Life set me on an alternate path to the one I had planned for myself, and eventually it led where I could not possibly have imagined going.

I believe every person has a destiny, that every circumstance and event furthers that destiny, even when all seems murky to the individual. Schopenhauer, in an essay entitled "On the Apparent Intention in the Life of an Individual," says that when one has lived long enough one can look back and see that all the circumstances of life, including obstacles and what

My Search for Healing

seem to be accidental events, are actually part of a master plan for one's life. That plan seems somehow to be built in—what is called *entelechy*, which Aristotle defined as the soul of the organized body. It signifies that which contains or realizes a natural end, whether of a process or a person. Entelechy suggests an agent inherent in the organism that directs the vital process toward the whole, or perfect realization of its inherent nature. A contemporary term derived from physics for this organizing principle is the *implicate order*. I have identified this as the Spiritually Evolving Life Force, which forms the basis of health and wholeness.

Working in an advertising agency, I quickly rose to a position of authority and status. Later, I became the owner of a graphic design studio on Madison Avenue, but I grew disillusioned and decided to quit commercial art. But what was I to do instead? I was reconsidering attending Columbia to obtain a Ph.D. in psychology when fate once again took a hand. I evidenced symptoms of ovarian cancer, which necessitated major surgery.

Because my father said I was the cause of my mother's death, when I was a child I assumed she had died giving birth to me. When I was fifteen, I discovered that she had died of cancer when I was a year old. However, since I was told that my birth was to blame for her death, by logical extension I then assumed she had died of reproductive-organ cancer. As a consequence of this line of reasoning, all of my life I had "known" that I would die of cancer when I reached the age at which my mother had died—a sort of propitiatory sacrifice, the biblical eye for an eye. I had accepted this inner dictum as absolute fact, so when my doctor informed me I quite possibly had ovarian cancer, it was right on schedule. Deeply poisoned by the years of ingrained guilt, my psychology and my biochemistry had melded to produce a disease. In the wake of which I understood that in response to the oft-repeated taunt, "You killed your mother," my

xvii

Healing Mind, Body, Spirit

child's psyche had set up a health-damaging quid pro quo. [*sth for sth*] Fortunately, the disease turned out to be endometriosis instead of the expected cancer. Two years later, I was diagnosed with breast cancer and experienced a spontaneous healing.

These two events taught me that the inner and outer worlds are not only inseparable but are in constant interaction. I wanted to know more about this, but I finally ruled out the academic pursuit of psychology. Not only would it have taken me from six to eight years to get the degree, but I was now convinced that psychology alone was not the answer to what I sought to learn. I knew there would one day come a field of study that would encompass both psychology and medicine—a psychobiology or a biopsychology at the time unimaginable for academia.

After I recovered from the surgeries, I left advertising for good to live by my own rhythms and discover my own truth. Soon thereafter, a synchronous series of events led to my employment by the Bollingen Series, which published the works of Carl G. Jung, the Swiss psychologist, then little known in this country and not then part of the academic curriculum in psychology. As I worked my way through the many volumes of his writings, previously unknown to me, I became fascinated by symbolism and alchemy; delved into Eastern philosophy mysticism, and yoga; explored the traditions of indigenous cultures; and began actively to interpret my dreams, which led to my discovery and practice of altered states of consciousness as a means of contacting the unconscious.

From Bollingen came the assignment to assist Joseph Campbell with preparation of his illustrated volume *The Mythic Image*. Unexpectedly, this work turned into a seven-year collaboration that plunged me deeply into the study of mythology, metaphysics, shamanism, symbolic art, ancient religions, goddess worship, magic, and the occult. In turn, this led me to the Tarot and astrology. Gradually I began to see that everything was connected to everything else, including healing, and that all

My Search for Healing

revolved around a spiritual center in the self. The divine was not out there somewhere, it was inside all of us.

In 1981, suffering from exhaustion due to overwork that had brought on a partial paralysis of my right arm, I spent three months in a German *kur-bad*, a rejuvenation clinic. There is no English language equivalent. Not a spa in the American sense, but not medical establishments either, the *kur-bad* became popular in the nineteenth century when "taking the waters" was a fashionable pursuit much favored by the European upper class. Whether private or state-run, the *kur-bad*, now a vital part of health maintenance for ordinary citizens and workers, is invariably situated at the source of natural mineral water springs. The word *bad*, literally bath, in the name of any German town indicates the presence of these healing waters, which are taken both internally and externally. Where the waters are thought to be particularly beneficial, whole towns are given over to these healing places, the world-famous Baden-Baden in the Black Forest and Bavaria's Weisbaden, once the seat of royalty, being two notable examples. Bad Bruckenau, where I went, was established by King Ludwig of Bavaria.

Different clinics have different specialties, such as post-operative, prevention, general rejuvenation for health-maintenance, weight-loss, or treatments for specific illnesses—cancer or chronic conditions like arthritis—but in all such towns there is always a large and beautifully landscaped *kur-park* for exercise and communing with nature, both essential components of the curative process.

At the clinic in Bad Bruckenau, I learned many healing methods, including the use of herbal teas, specific to each organ, for cleansing and restorative purposes; herbal baths for relaxation or energizing; hydrotherapy; deep muscle massage; and autogenous training, an advanced relaxation and imaging system that combines autosuggestion with guided imagery, an important part of the treatment. In this method, statements are

Healing Mind, Body, Spirit

tailored to implant in the subconscious an image of the condition desired for the body, as if it were actually in effect now. These phrases are said in timed repetitions while the mind is focused on the part of the body being addressed.

After leaving the clinic, I spent several months in Germany and there, while visiting a friend in Frankfurt, I discovered I possessed psychic abilities. This had been hinted at in my teens by a few startling experiences of precognition, but its sudden full activation felt as if I had spontaneously begun speaking in tongues!

Upon my return from this vividly experienced trip, I commenced to give Tarot readings and to practice astrology professionally. That there are influences we cannot see became absolutely clear. The truth of the concept that the mind is the intermediary between the everyday reality and that of the extraordinary was amply demonstrated.

On an extended trip to Mexico in 1982, I discovered I could heal others by the laying on of hands, and at the Copper Canyon, in a startling and totally unpremeditated demonstration, I was able, through the medium of drumming, to give healing "readings" to total strangers. This spontaneous experience, during which I felt I was being used as a medium by the Goddess speaking through me, heightened my interest in unseen powers. A year later, having become convinced through astrology that we each have a distinct pattern to live out—the knowledge of which could greatly aid in healing—I expanded my counseling practice to include a holistic form of psychology.

To serve my clients as holistically as possible, I also explored other natural means of healing: flower essences; crystals; aura reading; the therapeutic use of color, sound, and light; reflexology; body therapies such as Alexander Technique and shiatzu. I learned more about herbs, nutrition, and nutritional supplements.

My Search for Healing

By 1985, I had developed a mode of intensive therapy some clients found especially effective. This required my spending several days in succession with a single client. In order to facilitate this work, and to enable me to conduct group seminars, I rented a house in the Catskills. There I encountered the spirit of a four-hundred-year-old Native American *shaman* who taught me about healing methods he called "spiritual technology." He provided many important insights into the complex interactions of Nature and the human realm and gave me many direct healing sessions. Later, I discovered my house was situated directly over an old Indian burial ground. There followed, during an extended stay in Arizona, an intense period during which I received teachings from the invisible world, principally through dreams, visions, insights, and initiatory experiences.

In 1988, I developed post-polio syndrome, about which little is known and for which there is no effective treatment. Polio cuts off the nerve supply to the muscles; post-polio syndrome replays the original condition in midlife. So, though one may in childhood have escaped paralysis, it can occur later on. Determined not to become wheelchair-bound, I embarked on the use of the healing methods described in this book and, after not being able to walk for four months, regained mobility.

In 1991 I came down with chronic fatigue syndrome, a baffling illness some doctors think is purely psychological but, as anyone who has had it knows, it is quite physical in its effects. Thus, I had another opportunity to test the powers of self-healing. Within six months, I had overcome the condition, which can persist for years.

These then are the strands of my search for healing, of which this book is woven. I have learned that through the unfolding of our personal life drama we are led again and again into critical impasses that force us to seek resolution and healing. Healing is not an event but a *process*. It changes our evolving selves in a way akin to the transformations the alchemists worked, purifying matter with spirit to thus become whole. For this reason, I have chosen *transformation* as the focusing theme of this book.

While symptom removal may bring relief, true healing involves the whole self, not just the physical body. Mind, body, spirit are embedded in each other, feed and react upon each other. They cannot be separated. They function as one and must be treated as a whole, not a collection of parts.

Now, as I gather myself to the task of writing, these opening lines of a poem by Howard Moss, "The Pruned Tree," come to mind. They seem to me an apt metaphor for the transformational process called healing.

> *As a torn paper might seal up its side,*
> *Or a streak of water stitch itself to silk*
> *And disappear, my wound has been my healing,*
> *And I am made more beautiful by losses.*

M. J. Abadie
New York City
Thanksgiving Day, 1996

Introduction: The Inner Dynamics of Healing

Healing occurs when you align with the pure, positive energy that created the planet—and that keeps your heart beating and your blood chemistry normal. Healing occurs when you release <u>all</u> yourself to be well. Healing occurs when you're in harmony with your life's purpose and those who are meant to accompany you on this path. Healing occurs when you've created a sense of safety and security in your life. Healing is a major leap of faith in this culture.

— Christiane Northrup, M.D.
Women's Bodies, Women's Wisdom

Healing Mind, Body, Spirit

In our culture, there are two distinct types of healing. One is the standard, or *allopathic*, in which the practitioner, usually a medical doctor, intervenes directly by introducing medication that is designed to kill a specific bacterial or viral infection, or by performing surgery to repair or remove a damaged area. The other type of healing, so-called alternative medicine, is now coming to the fore due to increased interest. In this instance, the practitioner, whether homeopath, naturapath, acupuncturist, bodyworker, doctor of Chinese medicine, psychic, or other healer, seeks to help the afflicted to heal themselves.

Of course, there are instances when a doctor's intervention is necessary, such as in the setting of broken bones or the removal of invading foreign substances, which are beyond the individual's self-healing abilities. But it is widely recognized that many illnesses are "self-limiting," or will cure themselves if given time. According to Andrew Weill, M.D., the ratio is as high as 90 percent.

The truth is that ultimately *all* healing is *self-healing*. Medical doctors or surgeons, no matter how highly they regard their skills, must admit that the most they can do is make an accurate diagnosis and administer medicine or wield a scalpel. They must then rely on nature and the patient's inner resources to do the actual healing.

In order to influence effectively the imbalance that produces illness, the healing approach must reach into the *implicate order* of the person and reconnect to the original, unimpaired pattern of the *whole*. As illness is an expression on the physical plane of a disturbance in the field of the body-mind, its fundamental cause lies encoded in the relevant dynamics of each situation, especially those stemming from emotionally determined. Because the source is so deeply embedded, it is often necessary to direct healing efforts at the unconscious, or even the mythological or magical levels of existence.

However, the dominance of our scientific methodology has emptied medicine of mystery, mythology, magic, and spirit. Though these are rooted in concepts common to all cultures, doctors are taught to believe that the practice of medicine has nothing to do with such old-fashioned ideas. As a consequence of losing these vital connections, we find it difficult to grasp the true meaning of health, which means much more than the absence of physical infirmity or disease. *Health* derives from the Anglo-Saxon root that gives us *whole*, *hale*, and *holy*. *Medicine* comes from an ancient Indo-European root from which *remedy*, *meditate*, and *measure* also derive.

People in all ages and cultures have used various methods for refocusing consciousness and uniting themselves with their deepest and innermost selves, including music, dance, ritual, prayer, meditation, trance states, and physical agents such as the Native American sweatlodge ceremony. Through such means, they have called upon the energies inherent in themselves and their environments—including the animal and vegetable worlds and the cosmic or celestial realm—to heal. *Shamans*, such as Native American medicine men and other native healers, are as much religious leaders as they are doctors, treating physical and spiritual ailments as components of each other. Drawing upon energies both from the patient and from the community, the shaman heals by spiritually realigning the sick person with the natural order of being, at both a personal and cosmic level. This linking of the holy with the healthy is a basic tenet of traditional healing. Various types of "somatic" therapies—such as massage, acupressure, and reflexology—achieve their effects by being applied externally to the physical body to reach deep inside to the implicate order, where correction is made.

Healing Mind, Body, Spirit

In recent times, highly effective ways to utilize our inherent ability to refocus our consciousness have been developed. The most prominent are *breathing, relaxation, visualization,* and *meditation,* which form the central section of this book. Application of these methods can serve to harmonize discordancy and help us heal ourselves—mentally, emotionally, bodily, spiritually by connecting us with our inner patterns of health and wholeness.

Each person has a personal informational code in which genetic, glandular, emotional, and cognitive data are all stored. These data transmit information among themselves and with the environment. The *how* is an unknown, but there are recognized sources of information: the physical senses; intuition; emotions and feelings; the conscious mind; and, deeper still, the archetypes and myths of our heritage to which we resonate innately.

The mind is holographic in nature. Described by Karl Pribram in *The Holographic Hypothesis of Brain Function,* the model is based on the holograph, a three-dimensional picture produced by shining laser light through special film. Unlike ordinary photographs, the holograph has a unique characteristic. If you cut a holograph into pieces, each piece will contain the whole image of the photograph. A second characteristic is that, by shifting the angle of the plate, a holograph can be made to appear, disappear, and reappear.

Just as the holograph can reproduce the whole image from its tiniest part, what we call *mind* and *memory* are distributed throughout the entire organism—and possibly as part of the entire universe—in "nonlocal" fields. Larry Dossey, M.D., says that brainlike tissue is found throughout the body, making it difficult to follow a strictly local view of the functions of the brain. This concept indicates that we are much more "all of a piece" than the Western scientific, religious, and philosophic heritage suggests.

The Inner Dynamics of Healing

It is theorized that our bodies function in a holographic way as well, and that the implicate form principle is itself holographic in nature. Certainly this is indicated by some of the traditional and somatic therapies, a tenet of which is that one must look for the source of the dysfunction other than at the site of the pain or ailment, on the theory that some functions are not localized at specific sites but are distributed throughout the entire organism. At the very least, we are *connected* to ourselves at all points; we are not a collection of body and mind parts operating separately.

Recent experiments have shown that each of us contains an archive of holographic images—pictures of the past that continue to influence our emotions, behaviors, and health. These stored holographic pictures can influence or change our moods and feelings. Imprints from the past can impinge on you at any time, often without your knowing it is happening. You just *react*, but it is a reaction activated by an old pattern or memory.

The good news is that you can change your feelings—and even the cells of your body—radically, sometimes instantly, by using the relaxation, visualization, and meditation exercises and other tools in this book. This is because a picture we hold in front of our mind's eye can influence our bodies right down to the cellular level, often in an amazingly short period of time.

An example of this is the exciting new field of *psychoimmunology*, which is the study of the controlled use of imagery on the human body. Practitioners teach patients to visualize various healing scenarios. For example, *Omni* magazine detailed the following results of research done at Pennsylvania State University.

Wanting to test the claim that creative imagery can be used to combat cancer, Penn State psychologist Howard Hall taught a number of cancer patients self-hypnosis, a powerful relaxation tool. Then he instructed them in progressive relaxation techniques. The idea is that once the body is relaxed, the mind is open to utilizing the suggestions introduced by visualizations.

Next, he asked his patients to imagine their white blood cells—the body's first line of defense against any foreign or mutant cells that invade it—as "killers" attacking the cancer cells. Some imagined powerful, hungry sharks devouring their tumors. Children imagined a Pac-Man eating up the "bad" cells. They practiced their visualizations twice a day for a week, after which Dr. Hall checked the white blood cell counts.

The results were amazing. On average, the white blood cell count went *up* from 13,508 to 18,950, which showed that the patients' immune systems had rallied. Although some did better than others (which is to be expected considering individual differences both in ability and enthusiasm), Hall was convinced and said, "For some inexplicable reason, the mind can influence the body by changing the bio-chemistry of the blood."

Despite our new knowledge of brain chemistry, *mind* remains undefinable. Is the mind located in the brain? Is it distributed throughout the cells of the entire body? Is it "directed" by a universal Mind? Is it outside the body altogether, or is it something else entirely? No one knows.

However, there is a wide body of evidence suggesting the existence of a world organism based on a universal flow of information acting as its substructure. Physicist David Bohm calls this the *implicate order* and biologist Rupert Sheldrake hypothesizes *morphic fields*. Both of these ideas suggest interplay of all levels of existence, within ourselves and in the entire cosmos.

In view of this, and in an attempt to clarify terminology, I am proposing a new definition of the word *self*, redefining it as an acronym for *S*piritually *E*volving *L*ife *F*orce, represented typographically as SELF throughout the book.

Meant to encompass the totality of the human being, including the mind, body, spirit, and all their interactions, I use SELF to include *all* of the complex and multifaceted being that each one of us is. I believe that there is more to "mind" than brain, or

The Inner Dynamics of Healing

body cells, or their interactions. There is a spiritual dimension that cannot be ignored in a discussion of healing. No matter how you choose to identify it (as God, the Higher Power, the All One, etc.), this spiritual dimension is the creator of the implicate order, not only of ourselves, but of the entire cosmos.

As we explore that borderland where body, mind, spirit, soul, and earthly existence become One—where we merge not only with our whole selves but with the whole cosmos, and where substance and spirit interface—it is my hope that you will gain new insights into the unknown realms, what I have called "the invisible world," where true healing takes place.

It is not my intention, nor would it be possible, to offer a panacea or cure-all. We cannot say, "Take two meditations and one relaxation every four hours and cure yourself of whatever ails you." Healing is a vast and complex topic, and no single book can cover all aspects of it.

This book is not geared toward specific ailments, nor is it intended as a substitute for professional health care, conventional or alternative. Self-healing is an adjunct to, not a substitute for, these treatments. There is no denying that—despite its faults—when our Western medical technology works, it works very well indeed. However, it is my contention that while the interventions that characterize modern medicine can produce impressive results by eliminating many frightening symptoms almost instantaneously, such procedures may serve to short-circuit the deeper healing processes, which are necessary to living as whole persons.

By addressing healing in its broadest terms, this book aims to connect you to your own inner healing process, to encourage you to investigate all venues pertaining to your well-being, and to offer inspiration and, most of all, hope. To achieve this end, I will draw upon art, symbolism, mythology, and philosophy as well as the methods already mentioned. Healing is never purely physical; it involves the total organism, the *Spiritually Evolving Life Force*. To remove physical symptoms without resolving their underlying source is only to have illness return again in another form, or to produce a chronic condition. True healing is about becoming *whole*.

No matter what you want to heal at this moment, as you begin the healing process and devote yourself to it, you will experience the "magic" of connectedness. Making contact with your implicate order by recognizing that you are a *Spiritually Evolving Life Force* that contains within itself a perfect design can work wonders. Its effects may surprise you.

Remember, however, that healing is a *process*, not an event. Don't expect instant miracles. When you embark on self-healing, you step into a way of life, not merely a specific prescription for a particular condition or disease. Every individual is unique; what works for one may prove ineffective for another. Medical studies and research do not take that individuality factor into consideration, which is one reason conventional medicine, including mental health programs, often fails. It's up to you to make the effort to become acquainted with your own body, to face past traumatic conditions honestly, to assess your real needs, to act fearlessly and with confidence on the knowledge you gain, and, above all, to make a commitment to finding your personal way into healing. Treat your SELF with compassion, gentleness, patience, and respect, and you will be on the path to rejuvenation.

part one
Psyche and Soma

chapter one
The Mind-Body-Spirit Connection

The physician takes it for granted that disease germs exist as an integral part of the natural world. The metaphysician sees disease germs as the manifested result of anger, revenge, jealousy, fear.

~ Charles Fillmore
Atom Smashing Power of the Mind

◦ *Healing Mind, Body, Spirit*

Health issues are everywhere in the media today. Activists have garnered this extensive coverage by urging that more research is needed on a host of illnesses—AIDS, breast cancer, women's health, and, most recently, spinal cord injuries.

Daily we are exhorted to take better care of ourselves, to eat right, to exercise, to give up smoking, to moderate drinking. And, if health fails, we are encouraged to treat our conditions with vitamin supplements, herbal concoctions, nutritional correctness, and the like. Yet, after decades of "lite" and "lo-fat" products, and diet sodas, America is more overweight than ever.

Infectious diseases have been all but conquered in the West, but in their place we suffer from a host of chronic disorders. The scourge of cancer is as prevalent as ever.

The U.S. medical establishment, second in size only to the military establishment, is failing despite billions of dollars spent on research and a dazzling array of high technology equipment. The attempt to enslave Nature has backfired. Not only are Americans increasingly afflicted with a gamut of chronic illnesses—from diabetes and immune disorders to arthritis and heart disease—but depression and anxiety are rampant. Yet we do not look *within;* the very idea that so doing can help us is anathema in our fast-paced, performance-driven, bottom-line world.

We seek simple solutions to complex problems; yet, we refuse simplicity. Raised on expectations of instant gratification, we want a pill to make anything that bothers us go away NOW. Rather than interrogating *ourselves* to find out what the matter is, we look for some new guru to tell us what to do or for some new product such as fake fat to solve the problem. We look to the laboratory and the production line to cure what ails us.

Asking questions has never been encouraged and has sometimes been banned by our institutions of religion and medicine. Thus, we become dependent on and addicted to the latest panel

The Mind-Body-Spirit Connection

of experts who are presumed to know more than we do about our bodies, minds, and spirits. Failure to question—failure to ask the *right* question—plunges us into the morass. Psychologically, this is known as denial. We know something is wrong, but we refuse to acknowledge the problem.

In the myth of Parsifal, the young knight encounters a fisherman on the lake outside a magnificent castle. They strike up a conversation and the man sends him to the Grail castle, which is in a state of sorrow, for its lord, the Fisher King, is grievously ill with a wound that will not heal. Parsifal is ushered into a magnificent chamber, where the squire lies reclining on a stretcher. A feast is in progress and Parsifal witnesses marvels beyond belief. Exquisite food laid out on silver and golden platters magically appears, as does wine in jeweled goblets; beautiful women in wondrous gowns come and dance; flowers, music, sweet scents, delights of all kinds present themselves in an astonishing display. Though more than curious, Parsifal is a polite lad, who has been taught not to ask questions. Despite the revelry, the pain and sorrow caused by the lord's condition is evident. He is seen to bed by four fair maidens, but his sleep is troubled with terrible dreams. In the morning, he awakens—to an empty, silent, decaying castle. All is gone, lost for the want of a single question: "What ails you?" Parsifal leaves the Grail Castle an accursed man, reviled for ignoring the Fisher King's obvious condition. Later, after many adventures have freed Parsifal from reliance on social convention, he returns to the Grail Castle, asks the appropriate question, and the Fisher King is healed, the castle restored.

In *Cancer as a Turning Point*, author Lawrence LeShan says, "there is [a set] of questions…that *does* help clients increase their host resistance to the cancer. [What is] their most natural way of being, relating, creating?" What, in other words, would enable them to express themselves fully? How would they choose to live if, as LeShan proposes, "they adjusted the

Healing Mind, Body, Spirit

world to themselves instead of—as our patients generally have done—adjusting themselves to the world?"

Very often when LeShan asked his patients how they would change their lives given the opportunity to do so, they responded, "I don't know." He says, "The goal then becomes having them accept that this is the most important question at this stage of their life." He found that "mere acceptance of the question and a commitment to finding out out the answer" frequently had a positive effect on patients' immune systems.

Whether we must ultimately live with an illness or an infirmity does not preclude healing the *spirit*. Miracles do occur. LeShan speaks of cancer as being a turning point in a person's life. He says that the single thing that emerged most clearly was the context in which the cancer developed. In a large majority, "there had been, previous to the first noted signs of the cancer, a loss of hope in ever achieving a way of life that would give real and deep satisfaction."

We can, as traditional Cherokee believe, realize that sickness is intended as a purifying experience meant to return us to our path of destiny and spirit. Following that path is not easy. It is life's greatest challenge.

When the way was hard—money was often scarce and recognition seemed an impossible dream—I often rued my decision not to follow a conventional academic path. Had I known in advance the costs of being true to one's inner voice and the trials of making one's way outside society's mainstream—what Buddhists call the left-hand path—I might have taken the safer course and saved myself much anguish and travail. The left-hand path—or *individuation* in Jungian terms—is unforgiving and, once embarked on, impossible to forsake.

Many times I could have returned to a lucrative career in advertising and commercial art. I don't say I wasn't tempted by

The Mind-Body-Spirit Connection

an easier way, but at the end of the day my entelechy kept me going on a track whose direction and destination were still a mystery to me.

When I was twenty-five, I had the following conversation with the man I loved, who was intensely perplexed by my perpetual questing.

He: "What is it you are looking for?"
Me: "I don't know."
He: "What will you do when you find it?"
Me: "When I find it, I'll know what to do."

All these years later, I now know that I was seeking my spiritual center, where healing resides.

Joseph Campbell once astonished me by saying that I was one of only five or six true heroes he had ever known. Mystified by this unexpected accolade, I asked *why* he considered me a hero. He answered, "Because you never turned back, no matter what happened."

I make no claim of heroism for myself, but I do know that illness, trauma, failure, and defeat can draw out the best in us. Trauma of any kind, but especially illness, is—or can be—a call to the hero journey, which no longer is a journey of outward feats of braving danger and overcoming odds, but which instead is an inward quest to the center of one's being.

The first stage is withdrawal, and is mythologically represented as the descent into the underworld. When I was stricken with chronic fatigue syndrome, which was accompanied by a severe depression, and could hardly raise myself out of bed, it felt like I was going step by downward step into hell. As I lay bound to my bed, barely able to feed and sustain myself, beset constantly with thoughts of suicide, I felt that I was living the myth of the Sumerian goddess Innana, beautiful queen of the light-filled upperworld, who was summoned to visit her ugly sister, Ereshkigal, queen of the damned, in her hellish subterranean region.

Healing Mind, Body, Spirit

In her descent to the realm of her dark sibling, beautiful Innana had to pass through seven gates, at each of which she was stripped of some of her queenly raiment, until she arrived naked in the underworld and, having left all of her outward identity behind, was hung on a peg to die and rot in hell. I felt that I, too, was being forced to strip myself of all my garments—not clothing, but the trappings of regular life—in order to connect with my true identity; to learn my true purpose; to, in a sense, be able to go naked in the world, sustained by nothing other than who I am without artifice or pretense.

In *The Hero with a Thousand Faces*, Campbell says that once the local identifications of the persona and of society have been let go one is then "free to wander in the world as that essence," big with humanity as a pregnant woman is big with child. The life carried within waiting to be born is the new self, shorn, perhaps, but also tempered and made stronger.

Serious illness can be a means of stripping away the outer shell of unnecessary accumulations that have impeded us, though this is not always the case; the door is not always opened when opportunity knocks. Pain of any kind can bring opportunity, but, as philosopher Bertrand Russell observed, "Pain doesn't always ennoble. Often it merely crushes."

Do not be crushed by your pain. See it as an opportunity, a sharp tool to carve your way into your own spiritual center, where you will find the healing you seek.

Illness separates. When we become ill, we lose our means of livelihood, our beauty, our usual occupations, the sources of pleasure and satisfaction. Sometimes we lose our friends and find that family members avoid us. Without energy to cope with these losses, we must turn inward and descend into the netherworld of our being—there to confront our own dark sibling in the long and despairing dark night of the distressed but still unconquerable soul.

The Mind-Body-Spirit Connection

Before embarking on her journey to hell, Queen Innana had the forethought to call upon the water god Enki and make an arrangement with him for help should she fail to return. When the queen did not reappear, Enki fashioned, from the scrapings of his fingernails, two small mourners to grieve for the lovely Queen. He sent them down to the underworld to sit beside her as she hung mournfully on the stake, waiting to die. When the angry Ereshkigal saw these compassionate companions attending her bright sister and weeping tears of sincere sorrow for Innana's unfortunate condition, she relented and released Innana, explaining that she had only wanted to be acknowledged by her sister, recognized as being part of the family.

Ereshkigal is a metaphor for all that we have repressed, denied, left unshriven, hated, and failed to mourn, and for what shamed us, wounded us deeply, and has been left unfelt or unexpressed. These emotions sink deep into the unconscious, where they build a charge of negative power, which, finally, erupts into the upperworld, sometimes using the body as its vehicle of expression, sometimes the mind, sometimes both. When illness strikes, it is often because our dark sibling is trying to get our attention. I am here, she says, and we can no longer ignore her but must meet her long-denied demands for recognition.

We must fashion our own mourners out of the scrapings of our souls, to bear witness to our losses and travail and to give us the compassion we require. Too often, the gods of medicine and society have answered our desperate pleas with only drugs and surgery, or with platitudes, delivered without compassion or true caring.

LeShan comments that, although pathology must be taken into consideration, it is to be viewed in context, "as the process that blocks the perception and the expression of the individual's special song to sing in life; as the cause of his or her loss of contact with enthusiasm and joy."

Healing Mind, Body, Spirit

Some patients have negative reactions to the idea of singing their own song. They feel that it would be ugly and unacceptable, or impossible in this society, or so full of contradictions as to be useless. However, LeShan says that he has *never* seen anyone who, on finding his or her own special song and style, remained negative. *Never*. In addition, he says that "in every case the song was socially positive and acceptable."

Though it is natural to crave simple solutions to complex problems, ignoring our inner reality will not make it go away or be less complex. No drug has yet been invented that can substitute for one's necessary journey. Jung has said that neurosis is a substitute for legitimate suffering, and we must learn to legitimize our suffering by accepting it for what it can do for us, not by seeing it as the enemy invader. We must see the enemy and know that "he is us."

The trip to hell that is emotional trauma or serious illness can be a call to the hero journey with its message that persistence in the face of odds that at times seem overwhelming is the way to the inner self's proper powers. This is the boon promised by the quest, which the hero wins not only for himself but for his whole society through the ordeals of his trials and tribulations. Heroes are not only those who fight great battles, do daring deeds, run the marathon, or win Olympic gold medals. The hero journey is open to all. And it matters not if the hero is unsung, so long as each one is singing his or her singular song.

The hero's first work, according to Campbell, is the "retreat from the world scene of secondary effects to those causal zones of the psyche where the difficulties really reside," and "break through to the undistorted, direct experience and assimilation of...the archetypal images."

It is no accident that robust good health—the kind you take for granted and don't even have to think about—is referred to as "rude," as in the phrase, "Rude good health." To be perfectly healthy is to be in an unrefined state. Illness refines: it prunes,

The Mind-Body-Spirit Connection

trims, shapes, and reveals the powers that generate and sustain life; it is thus a form of initiation. It presents an opportunity to acknowledge that dark sibling self, so long repressed and ignored. To recognize its power is to enlist it in our aid. Purified by the ordeals we have experienced, we see clearly—often for the first time—what is of true value. Campbell notes, "all the life-potentialities that we never managed to bring to adult realization, those other portions of ourselves, are there; for such golden seeds do not die."

In the Eleusinian mysteries of ancient Greece, the initiate—as the last trial of his long initiation—was required to spend one night alone in "the valley of the shadow of death." When he emerged into the light from this frightful experience, he was shown a sheaf of corn—the emblem of the great mother goddess Demeter, who gives life to all on earth but also eats back the dead. It is said that the shock of recognition of this basic life–death power changed the consciousness of the initiate forever: having glimpsed the powers of creation, he was transformed.

This explains why the curing ceremonies of many indigenous peoples revolve around a reenactment of their creation myth. They believe that to realize one's place in the cosmic order is to find harmony and healing, to be renewed and refreshed, even reborn. The sixteenth-century alchemist-physician Gerhard Dorn wrote that, in order to heal, one must learn "from what one depends and to whom one belongs and to what end one has been created."

Our task, which is at the same time both simple and extremely complex, is to ferret out an approach that takes all of our "parts" into consideration—with gentleness and love. The maturation process is not one continuous, smooth transition from one stage of life to the next, but a continual process that is uneven at best. It is my contention that we all harbor multiple "selves," what I call simultaneous selves, made up of who we were at one time in our lives. Their fulfillment truncated for one reason or another, often by trauma but also by circumstance, they are split off from the whole. Yet, they continue to live as a "part" of us, influencing our behavior and our health.

We are usually at least dimly aware of our other selves, experiencing them as yearnings for lost youth, nostalgia for what might have been, feelings of dissatisfaction, regret, or, ultimately, as depression or illness, especially chronic ailments.

In my confrontation with chronic fatigue syndrome and its accompanying suicidal depression, I made contact with, and finally disgorged into full consciousness, one of these selves. In the throes of my illness, I understood that my desire to kill myself was actually a need to destroy an old source of pain, to kill the "me" who was still suffering from an old, unhealed injury. This understanding enabled me to redeem the buoyant, spontaneous young woman I was. Though I cannot today act as she did, I have reclaimed the feelings I had for so long been unable to experience.

Jung says,

> The serious problems of life...are never fully solved. If ever they should appear to be so this is a sure sign that something has been lost. The meaning and purpose of a problem seem to lie not in its solution but in our working it out incessantly.

We must seek avenues not only of comfort and consolation but of self-knowledge. While we are required to accept our natural limitations as human creatures, we are also able to probe our deepest natures to ascertain levels of our unrecognized human potential.

In terms of David Bohm's implicate/explicate orders, we are able to observe that every outer circumstance of our lives reflects an inner one. In Jungian terminology, the implicate is called

The Mind-Body-Spirit Connection

archetypal, and this archetypal field has the ability to affect our outer reality.

For healing to be effected, the relationship of these twin realities must be recognized and, if possible, brought to the level of consciousness. Explicate-form elements (the outer reality) are always in consonance with their correlative implicate, invisible patterns. Action or activity on either level affects the other. When the explicate order is affected by a properly tuned action, it resonates at the implicate level, and vice versa.

An example of an explicate action would be the introduction of acupuncture needles into the body at the invisible "meridians," which direct the flow of subtle energy on the implicate level. In the opposite direction, the seeking of dreams or use of meditation to activate the archetypal energy of the implicate order will ultimately affect the physical plane.

A brief example of how this can work is a dream I had that gave a specific prescription. In my daytime world, I had been having difficulty concentrating, and I could not figure out why. My mind just shut down and refused to admit any new information. Puzzling over this and suspecting everything from a brain tumor to some deeply recessed and unconscious psychological issue that I had somehow overlooked, I asked for help from the unconscious, or archetypal realm, as I was going to sleep. During the night, I had a dream in which I consulted a "doctor," who told me to begin immediately to take extra doses of vitamin C! There was no heavy symbolism to struggle to understand, no arcane images to be interpreted, just a straightforward remedy. When I rose, I took two thousand milligrams of vitamin C, another dose at mid-day, and another at dinner. I continued with this therapy, and in a short time my mental acuity had returned. Clearly, my body-mind knew what was causing the problem and what to do about it. This experience taught me a clear-cut and valuable lesson about trusting one's inner processes and the wisdom that arises from the intuitive realm.

Healing Mind, Body, Spirit

The implicate–explicate order system is like a Möbius strip, seemingly two-sided but actually a continuous loop. Whatever influences one side affects the other. Understanding this is basic to learning through nonlinear methods, such as intuition and dreams. These can effectively reconnect us to the state of balance that occurs when the flow of information between the implicate realm and its explicate manifest reality is unimpeded. Then, reunited with and released by our despised or repressed selves, freed of guilt and shame, open and free, we can embrace the totality of ourselves and, learning what is right for us, effect our healing.

chapter two
The Roots of Illness

It is becoming increasingly clear that what the shamans refer to as soul loss–that is, injury to the inviolate core which is the essence of a person's being–does manifest as despair, immunological damage, cancer, and a host of other very serious disorders.

— Jeanne Achterberg, "The Wounded Healer,"
in *Shaman's Path: Healing, Personal Growth and Empowerment*

~ *Healing Mind, Body, Spirit*

Illness does not occur in a vacuum, nor does healing. Both take place in the context of an entire life. Illness that manifests today may have been seeded anywhere along life's path, from earliest infancy to this morning. Illnesses are experienced in the dimensions of both body and psyche. Thus, healing—if it is to be effective—must take the whole person and the whole of his or her experience into consideration; healing must draw upon the information stored in our bodies and the deepest inner resources of the psyche.

The *roots* of illness lie in ourselves, and in our societies. They are both individual and cultural. They stem from who we are, what society sanctions or despises, the environment in which we live, what we value, and what we believe. "The enactment of the grand themes of our life drama structures our personality and character and becomes our physical constitution and its…illness," says Edward C. Whitmont, M.D., in *The Alchemy of Healing*.

Many of our ailments are behavior-related—heart disease; anorexia and bulimia; some cancers, such as lung cancer from smoking; emphysema; cirrhosis of the liver from drinking too much alcohol; melanoma from too much exposure to the sun; and sexually transmitted diseases, to name a few. Accidents, too, are often the result of our behavior or are caused by someone else's behavior.

Where does behavior come from? Behavior, especially compulsive or destructive behavior, does not just *happen to us*—it arises from the deepest psychic strata. It is a result of who we fundamentally are and how we react to the environment in which we live, to our life experiences, to the demands and expectations of society. No one holds a gun to the head of a workaholic or a smoker. Such behaviors serve psychological needs. Nicotine, for example, is known to numb feelings. Risky or careless behavior is a prime cause of both illness and accidents; those who indulge in such behavior are fulfilling inner needs and/or societal pressures. Behavior cannot be separated from the person whose behavior it is. Nor can it be separated from the society in which it occurs.

Stress is a major factor in illness; anywhere from 60 to 90 percent of visits to doctors stem from stress-related complaints. Stress is partly a result of behavior, but it is mostly a reaction to one's life circumstances. It, too, stems from the inner patterns of the individual. Everyone reacts to stress differently and handles stress well or poorly at different times for a variety of complex reasons. What upsets us when we are hungry or tired will not be a problem when we are fed and rested. Fear, anger, resentment, guilt, and anxiety are all inner stresses that show up as bodily illnesses such as ulcers, hypertension, skin eruptions, and other disorders.

Our behavior is often largely predicated on societal expectations and dictates. Men in the cutthroat business world are encouraged to be aggressively competitive, work long hours, and forgo self-nurturance. The deleterious results of this behavior are well known. Women, expected to be feminine and sexy while also holding down a job and raising children, are praised for denying their own needs. As a result, they suffer from a variety of illnesses, including those most difficult to diagnose. Seldom is our behavior purely *conscious* personal choice.

Some illnesses seem to come from out of nowhere, with no evident cause, such as chronic fatigue syndrome. Their source remains a mystery, but it, too, is rooted within the psyche and its environment. Other conditions appear to be genetic in origin, affecting only certain ethnic segments of the population. Yet the genetic malfunction skips around among those likely to be at risk. How to account for this is unknown. Theories like reincarnation have been put forth, and indeed these anomalies may represent some plan or purpose. Even infectious diseases do not infect everyone exposed to them. Sufficient numbers of people survived the bubonic Black Plague to repopulate Europe, and many attended the sick during cholera and other epidemic outbreaks without becoming ill. Why this is, no one knows, but the following story may give a hint to the wise.

A Westerner is teaching in Africa and, while attempting to explain the cause of malaria to his class of young boys, is greeted by bewilderment. Going over the lesson a second time, he reiterates that the mosquito is the carrier of the disease and that its bite can infect a person. The boys continue to stare blankly, and the teacher can see that his words aren't sinking in. Patiently, he once more begins a review of the facts, drawing a big, hairy mosquito on the blackboard. Suddenly, an excited lad shoots his arm up into the air and rises to his feet.

"But, sir," the boy questions agitatedly, "*who* sends the mosquito to bite the man?"

Those lucky few who have never suffered significant trauma or been seriously ill may perceive that illness is strictly physical or just "all in your head," but the truth is that no illness is only physical, nor is any merely "all in your head." The awareness that some conditions are "psychosomatic," or emotionally based, has led to the dismissal of certain ailments as not physical. But the person suffering a migraine headache as a result of emotional stress is every bit as physically affected as the person with a broken leg, and the emotional condition of the person with the broken leg may well be as responsible for his or her situation as is that of the migraine sufferer. Only when we recognize this connectedness will we be able to facilitate healing in a more generally effective way.

It is important to examine the pathology of diseases such as cancer that have clear physical symptoms; it is equally important to pursue identification of organic causes of illnesses currently not understood or able to be treated. However, it is of paramount importance—especially for those who are living with illness—to listen to the whole story, not just to look at the X-rays and the laboratory test results. We cannot understand the illness, or find its cure, unless we understand the person who has the illness. We may one day discover that what cures cancer in one person will not cure the same cancer in another person, because of the difference in innate proclivities and life experience.

Depression is a case in point. Usually treated as a purely emotional/psychological condition, depression can actually result from allergic response, chemical sensitivity, or an imbalance of neurotransmitters, which can be alleviated by medicine. Depression can be a *symptom* of a physical imbalance. Equally, a physical impairment can be the symptom of an underlying problem such as depression.

In the great Hermetic sixteenth century, a physician first studied astrology, magic, and numerology. Paracelsus, a physician known for his ability to heal by psychic means (*thaumaturgy*), wrote that "Magic is a teacher of medicine preferable to all the written books," and by magic he meant "power that comes direct from God," or contact with the whole: *whole=holy*. He believed that health derived from harmony between the person and nature, that man is a microcosm of the One, the macrocosm.

Nostradamus—another sixteenth-century physician, and author of the famous and astonishingly accurate *Centuries* prophecies, which are still studied today—was both an astrologer and a scientist. Unlike today, when the straitjacket of academic discipline and rigorous separation of fields of study have been imposed on the inquiring minds of students and professionals alike, in earlier times there was no distinction between magic and science, nor between astronomy and astrology.

But when, in the seventeenth century, body and soul were separated from each other by René Descartes's famous dictum, "I think, therefore I am," physical processes began to be compared to mechanics; psychic experience was dismissed as a fuzzy flight of fantasy, a product of the imagination. It was classified by definition as an activity indulged in only by the weak, emotionally immature, or mentally infirm—a definition most often applied to women by men and male doctors.

Ever since this famous mind-body split occurred, we have been told by our doctors, when they are baffled and cannot diagnose, "You're just imagining things." This, in effect, blames the patient for getting sick. Too busy to be bothered, our doctors fail to listen to the patient's whole story and thus perpetuate the difficulty instead of ameliorating it.

In the scientific paradigm that we inherited from the European scientific revolution, body and mind are related only by direct cause and effect and are to be regarded as two separate entities. I drop a ball and it hits the ground. That's cause and effect between two separate entities. But what about the following scenario? I absentmindedly set a heavy can of tomato juice on top of the refrigerator so that it overhangs the juncture with the door, and then, when I open the door, it falls in such a way that the sharp rim hits my bare foot and breaks all the bones across the arch—on a Thanksgiving Day when I am hosting an obligatory party against my will and am fed up with listening to people argue? My "freak" accident and immediately swollen foot ends my participation in the unwanted social event and sends everyone home. Cause and effect, or body-mind connection?

Attempting to divorce the physical from the mental and emotional is like trying to consider the fingers separate from the hand. But in the cause-and-effect model, illnesses are either/or. They are physical or mental, with no connection between the two. People with maladies diagnosed as organic are given respectful treatment; those with ailments not seen to have an organic cause are dismissed as neurotic. The actual experience of illness defies that dichotomy.

For example, when I was recovering from the surgeries connected to having endometriosis, I realized that this illness was putting me in touch with my father's inexplicable rage against me. Once out of its reach, I had attempted to shrug off his animosity as no longer important or threatening. But the severe childhood abuse had been somatized deep in my psyche, even-

The Roots of Illness

tually manifested as physical illness. The illness gave me the opportunity to reconnect with that hurt part of myself long stored away. Having a part of my living tissue cut out of me seemed to serve as a symbolic reference point. What had previously been cut out of my life on the emotional level was now visible on the physical level. And it was my reproductive organs that were affected, echoing my childhood belief that my mother had died giving birth to me. I was also able to see my disease as symbolic of what emotionally was influencing me in inappropriate ways and needed to be self-excised. During my long recovery period, I began to contact deep layers of my body memories, activating a consciousness that was so fundamental as to be cellular: the body remembers not only what has happened but also how to heal it.

Endometriosis is the second leading cause of infertility and is a terrible source of pain for countless women. Research by Dr. Andrea Rapkin, M.D., of the UCLA School of Medicine, has shown a high incidence of abuse in these patients. It is not totally clear whether early or ongoing abuse is a specific factor in endometriosis, but emotional, physical, and sexual abuse abound in the life histories of women with chronic pelvic pain. Physician Margaret Caudill of the Division of Behavioral Medicine at Harvard Medical School says that these patients' descriptions of their pain "mirrors the effects of the psychological trauma they've experienced. They feel out of control. They hurt all the time. They say nobody believes them." She goes on to say that grappling directly with their abuse can lessen the pain.

Illness requires withdrawal. Solitude gives us a chance to process what is happening to us, to understand and put it into perspective. And this enlarges us spiritually. Dr. Theodore Rubin says, "If one is sick and must withdraw, then withdrawal is healthy...to gather strength so as to be able to emerge." It is only when you are alone that you can devote sufficient attention to your own healing, without having to consider the needs of others. Ill people were once moved into seclusion in order to cope with their ailments. Today we consider isolation to be old-fashioned and unliberated. The most seriously ill, those in intensive-care units, are monitored twenty-four hours a day by noisy machines in brightly lit rooms attended by a phalanx of medical personnel; they are never allowed to be alone or quiet.

Time alone gives us the opportunity to receive guidance from our Higher Selves, to contact the healer within, to delve into our personal mysteries, to come to terms with who we are and where we are going in life. In my case, the onset of endometriosis was the end of my career in advertising and the beginning of my metaphysical search, which in turn led me to working with Joseph Campbell. It signaled a major and lasting life change and brought me closer to my own truth.

Our illnesses, wherever they may come from, call us to *ourselves*—our symptoms, whether minor or severe, are messages from our deeps; they want us to reorient ourselves to, if you will, our souls. When we refuse to give ourselves time to regenerate and to process ourselves into the new stage of life signaled by illness or distress, we build up to toxic levels that can erupt in more illness later. Morris Berman, in *The Re-Enchantment of the World*, says, "Soul is another name for what the body does."

Many of us hate our bodies. Instead of glorying in the wonder of our selves and appreciating our bodies for the marvelously efficient, automatically functioning entities that they are, we find fault with every conceivable aspect. Instead of accepting with gratitude the uniqueness Nature has given us, we criticize and critique our physical selves.

This self-hate of our physical appearance can often lead to serious emotional illness, especially for women. Our rejection of our bodies spawns a host of other problems, such as low self-esteem and lack of self-confidence. These then intertwine with our bad body image to create a cycle of negativity that causes many of our ailments.

Although our bodies smoothly perform the vast majority of our physical functions without our conscious awareness—storing energy converted from food, processing and eliminating toxic wastes, breathing, re-energizing us while we sleep, yawning when more oxygen is needed, avoiding danger by reflex actions, and more—we continue to despise them, bewailing their configurations, denying their needs, discrediting their value, denigrating their beauty. Why is this?

We are taught to look down on our "animal" side. The very word *animal* is used in a pejorative sense—"Don't be such an animal!" or "How disgusting—you're acting like an animal." In truth, animals never act in the ways we characterize as being "animal." Only humans do. Acceptance of our bodies is necessary to healing them. What is your relationship with your body? Do you resent or demean your animal self; find natural functions disgusting; deplore your body's size, shape, or condition? Are you riddled with shame and guilt about your body? Do you try to avoid looking at it? If so, you are falling prey to the fallacy that there is a fundamental split between your biological animal self and your rational mind. This split keeps you from experiencing yourself as one single and unified human being—in short, from acknowledging your SELF.

This widespread alienation of people from their bodies and, consequently, from their animal natures has led many of us into self-abuse and neglect and is one of the roots of illness. Your body is not just a convenient storage bin for your brain; it is the home of your spiritual self. One does not exist without the other. The Hawaiian tradition of Huna teaches that we are composed of three "beings" that interpenetrate each other. One is the animal self; the second is the mental self; the third is the spiritual self. Each needs and serves the other in harmonious cooperation within the whole.

Healing Mind, Body, Spirit

When what is merely "natural" to us is unacceptable in the eyes of those in power over us, we push down our natural impulses to live authentically, driving the negative force into our very flesh and blood where it festers like the uncleaned wound it is. Illness is the price we pay for suppressing the true expression of our SELF.

The truth is that what we hate isn't just the body, it's ourselves, inside. Where do you get your self-image from? This may sound trite, but you get it from *yourself*. Unconsciously, perhaps, but nonetheless so. All your life you have been telling yourself what you think of yourself. At first, when you were very young, you absorbed what others said and thought about you and took it as the gospel truth. Later, you continued to play these "parent tapes," even while consciously rejecting their input. Your view of your self is a product of your opinions about yourself.

A lifetime of repetition has forged a self-opinion you now must either live with, suffering the painful consequences, or begin to change. This is called *cognitive reframing*. One of LeShan's cancer patients put it this way:

> What I hear you saying is that I have lived my life as if I bought my clothes off the rack. They fitted pretty well, but were standard issue. And that if I want to set my immune system an example I have to start living my life as if I were having my clothes made especially for me by a top-level couturier—clothes and a life that is designed specifically for me, not for someone approximately my size who wants to fit in with everyone else and be wearing whatever is fashionable at the moment. That if I really get committed to this, then it will be as if my immune system looks up, says, "Oh, this specific individual is worth fighting for. Why didn't you say that before?" I've got to set my body an example by taking care of me and gardening who *I* am, not just adjusting myself to whatever is on the clothing rack of life.

The Roots of Illness

Fortunately, change is possible. You can tune in to your muscles and find out just what is *somatized*—stored in there. You may find old pain you no longer even remember consciously. Be loving and gentle with yourself, not critical or judgmental. Open yourself to what you may find when you ask your tense muscles what bad memories they are holding. You may recall times when you felt humiliated or powerless, wanting to act to protect or avenge yourself, but unable to do so for one reason or another—usually because you *were* weak and powerless.

Many of us live in a state of perpetual tension, our muscles hardened into rigid and painful sets. Psychologist Wilhelm Reich called these immobilized muscles "body armor." The tension resulting from the "fight or flight" syndrome remains in the body, unreleased by action, holding energy in the muscular contractions. The original source may be years in the past. Reich's therapy was to knead these stiff muscles to relax them, and a by-product was the release of *emotional pain*, produced at the time of the original assault on the person's sensitivities and stored along with the physical tension. During the course of body therapy, many people reexperience the original pain of the event that created the body armoring. Some, at the sudden release of long-stored energy, burst into tears or express the held-in emotion in other dramatic ways.

Over the years, I have worked through many of my own muscular tensions, but one stubborn area remained chronic in my right shoulder, which had a "trigger point"—a spot that, under stress, is capable of producing excruciating pain. I had consulted various therapists, done body work, and had chiropractic treatments, but even if I got some relief temporarily, the chronic tension soon returned. On three occasions I experienced unremitting, debilitating pain for ten days straight.

For a time I attributed it to long hours spent typing or at a desk or drawing board. Finally, I made a startling connection. Feeling my way back along the chains of memory, I tried to find the original experience and its emotional content. It occurred when I was twenty-one.

My stepmother, with whom I had remained in contact out of compassion, asked me to care for three of her five small children for two weeks so that she could attend her terminally ill father. I agreed, even though it meant rearranging my apartment and my life. During the second week, in the middle of the night, the youngest boy had an attack of appendicitis and had to be hospitalized for immediate surgery. On the way to the hospital, he told me he had often had these painful attacks *but had never been taken to a doctor*. I was appalled and furious at this neglect of the child, and in the morning when I telephoned my stepmother to inform her of the situation, I told her so in no uncertain terms.

A great deal of acrimony ensued, during which I had to fend off my father's hysterical demand that the hospitalized child be flown home at once. The next day, my stepmother arrived on my doorstep and accused me of being responsible for the child's need for emergency surgery. So that she could be comfortably nearby and visit the boy while he was recovering, I installed her in my apartment with the children and moved in with a friend. A couple of days later, without telling me, the doctor, or the hospital staff, she took the boy out of the hospital and disappeared from my apartment. The doctor discovered the boy's absence when he made his rounds and telephoned me at work. I rushed home to find all traces of her and the children gone. The surgeon had warned of grave risks should the boy not receive proper postoperative care. I had no idea where my stepmother was, but I assumed she was on her way home, a long drive.

Knowing the child would need immediate medical care, and not at all certain his mother would realize this, I had no choice but to telephone my father and explain the situation. It was unpleasant to say the least, but my father had the sense to realize his wife had put his son in grave danger and promised to see to the rectification of the situation when they arrived home.

A week later I received a legal document, sent by registered mail, formally disowning me, stating in legal terms that I was no longer my father's daughter. The accompanying letter filled with accusations against me made it evident that, in order to avoid my father's wrath at her unwarranted action, which jeopardized the child's life, my stepmother had manipulated the situation by concocting a story about me. Exactly what she invented I will never know. My conscious reaction was "good riddance."

Soon thereafter, I suffered such a stiffening in my shoulder muscles that my head was literally pulled down onto one shoulder at a right angle. This went on for weeks until finally I realized I was in a seriously bad way. A friend recommended an osteopath, a kind and gentle man who worked with me for several sessions before the "kink" was removed. He told me that had I waited even another day before seeking treatment, he would have had to put me in traction in a hospital.

For years, the condition persisted as a chronic problem, causing me much pain and tension, until I finally made the connection: I had "shouldered" responsibility that was not mine and then been "stabbed in the back" for my efforts. This realization enabled me to dissolve the somatized painful emotion that had collected in my musculature. Even now, as I tell you this in the hope that my experience will help you to heal your pain, in body and mind and spirit, tears well up in my eyes. But they are tears of release.

Along with unacknowledged or repressed grief and emotional pain, feelings of worthlessness are a principal root of all illness. In her book *Healing Mind, Healthy Woman*, Alice Domar says, "Self-esteem is a women's health issue," but it is no less an issue for everyone. When we think of ourselves as being unimportant or unlovable, or are filled with guilt and shame, we don't take proper care of ourselves. We may delay necessary medical care, fail to eat properly, use inadequate protection from the elements, take unnecessary risks, not bother to learn about and practice good nutrition and regular preventive health measures.

The antidote is to <u>honor ourselves</u>—body, mind, and spirit—and to make an unwavering commitment to taking care of ourselves. When we honor our bodies, we honor our spirits, and when we hold our spirits in honor, we see our bodies as sacred. When we honor the SELF, we support our innate capacities for self-repair and regeneration. I like the idea of making a covenant with ourselves to honor ourselves. In *Honoring the Self*, Nathanial Branden expresses this beautifully:

> To honor the self is to be willing to think independently, to live by our own mind, and to have the courage of our perceptions and judgments.
>
> To honor the self is to be willing to know not only what we think but also what we feel, what we want, need, desire, suffer over, are frightened or angered by—and to accept our right to experience such feelings. The opposite of this attitude is denial, disowning, repression—self-repudiation.
>
> To honor the self is to preserve an attitude of self-acceptance—which means to accept what we are, without self-oppression or self-castigation, without any pretense about the truth of our own being, pretense aimed at deceiving either ourselves or anyone else.
>
> To honor the self is to live authentically, to speak and act from our innermost convictions and feelings.
>
> To honor the self is to refuse to accept unearned guilt and to do our best to correct such guilt as we may have earned.
>
> To honor the self is to be committed to our right to exist, which proceeds from the knowledge that our life does not belong to someone else's expectations. To many people, this is a terrifying responsibility. To honor the self is to be in love with our own life, in love with our own possibilities for growth and experiencing joy, in love with the process of discovering and exploring our distinctively human potentialities.

part two
Transformations of Healing

chapter three
Healing: An Alchemical Process

The greatest treasure comes out of the most despised and secret places.... This place of greatest vulnerability is also a holy place, a place of healing.

— Albert Kreinheder
Body and Soul: The Other Side of Illness

Carl Jung devoted ten years to the study of alchemy. The two magnificent volumes produced as a result of his research inspired widespread interest in alchemical symbolism, especially in the psychological community.

Previously, the popular conception was that the alchemists were either deluded fools or money-mad charlatans attempting to turn lead into gold in their secret laboratories. When he began to research the alchemical texts, Jung, in compliance with the mindset of Western science still dominant today, thought alchemy "stuff and nonsense." However, by interpreting the arcane formulas and symbolism metaphorically rather than literally, Jung's exhaustive study showed him that alchemy was "the historical counterpart of [his] psychology of the unconscious." He observed that the alchemists' methods were "sufficient to activate the unconscious and, through the power of imagination, to bring into being things that apparently were not there before."

Jung's insights into the baffling symbolism of the alchemists enabled him to erect a psychological model that can serve as a guide to the stages and processes of the spiritual transformation that underlie healing.

In the final analysis, all healing is a spiritual process, and the evolution of our spirituality involves a process of *transformation*.

In alchemy, a major phase was the *nigredo*, or blackening, which followed upon several stages of breakdown. In old texts, this was pictured as an old and dying king, or a youth laid out on his deathbed. We can view illness as the *nigredo*—not the beginning but the turning point. From a psychological perspective, the experience of the *nigredo* is analogous to the encounter with the dark sibling.

Illness, whether physical or emotional, presents the opportunity to prune away the dross that prevents us from living fully. First, there is the experience of "blackening"—of defeat, loss, humiliation, fear, anxiety. Once, however, that we progress beyond the "Why me?" stage of confronting painful experience, the occasion arises to ask of ourselves the question, "What ails thee?" from a deeper perspective than that of medical diagnosis. We can ask, "What does this mean?" "How can this experience help to make me whole?" or "What is here that will enhance my spiritual growth?"

Called the "Great Work," alchemy was based upon the idea that there slumbers in matter "a divine secret." To unveil it was to produce the *lapis philosophorum*, or philosopher's stone, from the *prima materia*—lead, or "base," matter, symbolic of the dark and hidden forces of Nature. The characteristics of the *prima materia* are that it is common and readily available; it is considered revolting or disgusting; it has many forms but only one essence; and it is omnipresent. Psychologically it represents what we have debased by rejection or repression; it is what we consider unacceptable in ourselves, which in Jungian terms is known as the "shadow."

The *prima materia* was put into a retort, or the crucible, and subjected to intense heat. Being dissolved in its own juices, so to speak, led to its transformation into the *lapis*. In other words, the ugly material stuff contains within itself the gold of the spirit.

Though the medieval alchemists worked in a laboratory with chemical ingredients, it was their aim to purify themselves, to transform the personality, and by so doing to effect a similar transformation in the raw material of nature. The burning away of impurities in the furnace was to be seen as symbolic of the alchemist himself undergoing a purification spiritually, in order to release the "higher" in himself. Said Jung, "There is no doubt that the goal of the philosophical alchemist was higher self-development, or the production of...the *homo major*, or what I would call individuation." The end was not only personal salvation, it was intended to "cure" the impurities in matter itself and release the Divine Energy into the world.

~ Healing Mind, Body, Spirit

Paracelsus, one of the great masters of alchemy and a physician, said that each disease "bears its own remedy within itself," that "Health must grow from the same root as disease."

This conception is at the center of homeopathy and forms the basis for treatment. Homeopathic remedies are made of substances that in large doses would produce the illness they are—in extremely dilute form—prescribed to cure. This understanding that the curative agent is "sleeping" in the very matter that caused the problem in the first place is the basis of transformational healing.

A Jungian analyst, Arnold Mindell, leads his patients to exaggerate their symptoms—wallow in their misery—until a breakthrough occurs. This is an experience familiar to me and to many people who have suffered serious illness of either an emotional or physical nature. It is called the "healing crisis." Illness is the crucible. It serves to amplify the distress, turn up the heat so to speak. One gets worse—and often gives up all hope—before, usually quite suddenly, there is relief: we see the light at the end of the tunnel. As Joseph Campbell remarks, "One thing that comes out in myths is that at the bottom of the abyss comes the voice of salvation. The black moment is the moment when the real message of transformation is going to come. At the darkest moment comes the light."

The first step in the alchemical transformation is the gross matter, or the illness. The second, the closed retort, or crucible, which is the isolation of the ill person, who is separated from society and the ordinary course of life, the better to concentrate attention on the self. The third is the dissolving, or reduction to the original state. At this last stage, which is closest to the implicate order, we are often given clues in dreams.

For example, during a severe writer's block, which was accompanied by excruciating pain in my left arm and shoulder, I had a vivid dream in which an all-powerful figure, a "doctor," told me he was going to inject a substance into my brain that would rejuvenate the brain cells by rearranging them into another pattern. The dream showed me that the reason I was stuck was that I was unwilling to let go of the original structure, which was the source of the problem. I had to have my brain cells rearranged—let go of the old and unworkable pattern in order to be able to rethink the problem and reach resolution.

Illness often occurs when we are stuck in life. It can serve to liberate us from circumstances that are preventing our emergence into a new phase more suitable to our needs and aspirations, leading us into our larger selves. Many, like LeShan's cancer patients, have called their illnesses "a turning point," saying they discovered joy and awareness through their encounter with illness, especially life-threatening kinds. An illness, even a relatively minor one, can lead to a realization that something in our lives needs to be restructured to better ourselves in some way.

The hero journey can be viewed from an alchemical perspective as, through his trials and tribulations, the hero undergoes a process of transformation that awakens him to the divine secret in Nature. When we begin seriously to explore our healing potential, we open a magical door to the unconscious, to the implicate order.

On the journey formidable obstacles are encountered, but help is received from those treated with respect and honor. The demons, fearsome beasts, and strange, unrecognizable beings—often ugly and threatening—that must be met and overcome are our psychological projections. Sometimes an animal is encountered, representative of the instinctive realm, who renders aid when danger threatens, or reveals the concealed path.

Often there is an old and repulsive crone who solicits assistance. When it is given, she turns into a delightful maiden of extraordinary beauty who showers the hero with her favors and gifts. However, if he is revolted by her gross appearance and refuses the aid she requests, he finds his way is blocked by new and treacherous obstacles.

The ugly crone is the Goddess who tests the hero at every turn, Mother Matter from whom all earthly things are formed. In Greek mythology, she is Hera, Queen of Olympus, or Demeter, Mother Earth. But the Great Goddess also has a dark side, the Terrible Mother who eats back her dead children and promotes death and decay in order to bring forth new life. Jung called this side of Her *chthonic* in reference to the underworld where Ereshkigal resides, and psychologist Erich Neumann describes "the realm of the Mothers" as that most mysterious of life forces inherent in the matter from which the Earth and all on it are made.

The hero must encounter the Goddess in her unloveliest of forms, for the processes of Nature from which new life arises—death and decay, decomposition, malodorous waste—are disgusting to us and we turn our eyes away from or try to hide or deodorize them. Yet, these are the *prima materia* from which the divine *lapis* is distilled.

When the hero has learned to face the terrible Goddess with compassion and without flinching, she reveals her beauty and bounty. He is wonder-struck at the blissful revelation, healed of all his infirmities, shorn of his woes, lifted out of his confusion into understanding, transformed from a callow youth immersed in social dependencies and obligations to an independent individual who has incorporated the divine nature within himself. In a word, he has received enlightenment.

Like the hero, the sick person must confront demons and overcome them, must confront the dark Goddess within the psyche and recognize the beauty inherent in the apparent ugliness. Our innermost private self, that place where we hide the things we find gruesome or unacceptable must be honored with our compassion. Then, our inner demons turn into helpers and lead us into healing and health and we see revealed the bright face of the Goddess of life. Through facing our darkness, we enable the light of the spirit to shine through us, transforming it into the gold of spiritual realization.

Some years ago, I was with Joseph Campbell attending a theatrical performance staged by his wife, the dancer-choreographer Jean Erdman. A trilogy called "Moon Mysteries," based on the work of W. B. Yeats, one of the pieces was the story of a lame man and a blind man who were on the road in search of a magic well that healed. The lame man rode upon the back of the able-bodied blind man, directing him. When these journeyers reached the magic well, they encountered the spirit of the well who challenged them.

"Would you rather be cured or saved?" asked the spirit.

"Cured," the blind man said promptly and received his sight.

But the lame man opted for salvation and went whirling off in a wonderfully antic, joy-filled, one-legged dance.

The entire performance was deeply affecting and at some point during it Campbell and I had linked hands. When the lights came up at intermission, he squeezed my fingers and said softly, "Would *you* rather be cured or saved?"

"Cured," I said with no hesitation. "Which would you choose?"

"I want to be saved," said he.

"*Saved?*" I replied in amazement, for I thought he had long since left behind all notions of heavenly salvation.

"Yes. I have always wanted my name writ large in the book of heaven."

As I reflect on that experience, I have no doubt that he got his wish, but the question arises: must we choose between being cured and saved? Or are these two concepts inextricably linked? Perhaps it is necessary to draw a distinction between being "cured" and being "healed." And perhaps being healed is more akin to being saved than is a mere cure, or the removal of physical symptoms. The need for healing draws forth the spiritual energy that engenders wholeness. And to be made whole is to be saved. As Jung says in relation to the therapeutic work, "The labours...are directed towards that hidden and as yet unmanifest 'whole' man, who is at once the greater and the future man."

Once I believed art to be a key to healing. I spent countless hours in museums, galleries, and libraries absorbing the history of the world's art and studying the lives of artists. I pursued literature and poetry, and attended theatre, opera, and ballet performances. Though subsequent experience taught me that art, while *a* great healer, is not the only one, I made an important discovery through the study of art and the lives of artists: the *becoming* of the artist is a transformative spiritual process analogous to the transformative experience of healing. In addition, it was through art that I encountered symbolism, which lies at the heart of the alchemical transformational process that healing is.

It has been said that art is what results from the artist's inner struggle. Thomas Mann said, "One does what one is and art is truth—the truth about the artist." Thus is authentic art created out of the transformative fires of the growth experience of becoming an artist. Talent aside, the *process* of becoming an artist affects not only the end product, the "art," but it also (and perhaps more importantly) affects the artist, as does the subject matter chosen for the expression of the SELF. In a profound and transformative interaction, each acting upon the other in the complex mingling of inner and outer realities, artist and subject matter fuse and become one.

So it is with all of us. It does not matter what work we do as we practice the art of living our lives. What we choose to focus our attention on shapes us as much as we shape it.

I believe all *authentic* art is an attempt to fuse inner and outer realities. We might even say that art *is* alchemy. Though some artists, like Vincent van Gogh and Mozart, are destroyed in the fires of their creative vision, this process of self-transformation is similar to the alchemists' efforts to bring forth the *lapis philosophorum*, a process meant to purify both the substance and the alchemist who performed the work. What is sought is not the common gold of the marketplace but the gold of philosophy, or, to quote Campbell, "gold, in other words, such as only art bestows, through its transfiguration of the world as commonly known."

A telling example is that of a highly successful playwright-screenwriter, who, in the wake of a heart attack in his mid-fifties, publicly lamented that, having devoted his talent to insubstantial popular froth, he feared he would never be able to write anything of true artistic significance. By pursuing commerce rather than art, he had refused the process of transformation that might have made him great—and suffered a "broken" heart as a result.

In the transformational process of healing, which is not unlike the alchemist's and the artist's, we achieve the desired end by *submitting* to the requirements of our authentic selves. Our soul-directedness, or *entelechy*—what I call the "internal imperative"—is like an inborn compass that serves to keep us on the course that will fulfill who we truly are, without the societal and personal-traumatic overlays. Physical illness and psychological trauma indicate that we are off-course and must make the necessary corrections to return ourselves to the state of balance that is health. They force us to come to grips with this inward reality.

I select the word "submit" carefully to imply a definite *willingness to yield to our own inner process*. Unless we are willing to submit to the larger order of ourselves, which is the bearer of healing, little will be attained. This conscious surrender never comes without a concomitant struggle: hence, *submit*. It is this very stance that promotes the healing we seek.

~ Healing Mind, Body, Spirit

This larger order is the inner dynamic of who we really *are*—not who we suppose ourselves to be based on the expectations of ourselves, our parents, our teachers, our religious leaders, our society. Each person carries his or her true reality within, and this reality is always seeking contact with our conscious minds. It works through many channels, including our dreams and experiences that seem to be random or merely happenstance, such as accidents and illness.

In this context, in *The Alchemy of Healing*, Edward C. Whitmont, M.D., says,

> Some form of assimilation by personal or vicarious surrender to the entelechy of the Self-field is then required, or even forced upon us by illness or relationship problems. These are bent upon connecting and reconnecting us to the implicate essence and its reordering stream of information, psychologically and/or physically.

The ingrained habit of separating mind and matter, sanctioned by our current scientific worldview, has grave consequences. To regard our illnesses as if they are fundamentally separate from our own essential nature is to court disaster. True healing can only take place within a holistic model. Anything else sanctions the abuse of ourselves and our planet.

What we think and feel affect how we are physically, and bodily states work their way out through our emotions and thoughts. Homeopaths and other "alternative" practitioners know that diagnosis and treatment must include the patient's personality, temperament, emotional state, and spiritual needs. Speaking of homeopathy, Dr. Whitmont says, in *The Alchemy of Healing*,

> The choice of medicine is always approached in terms of bio-emotional wholeness, hence implying an equivalent origin of the illness. Diagnostic indications for potentially beneficial

medicines always have to include the patient's temperamental and emotional state....I noted the similarity of the homeopathic approach to the alchemical viewpoint. The alchemical process also requires an integration of molecular-based substance and the psychodynamically arising complexes.

Unlike those imbued with the Western scientific worldview, the alchemists were keen observers of the transformational process that occurs both in the manifest world (the explicate order) and in the invisible world (the implicate order). For the alchemists, if the work were to be effective, it was essential that there be no separation of spirit, body, mind, and substance. The transformative process required complete integration, total emotional and psychological honesty, and a genuine transformation of the laborant. To fail in this endeavor was to fall into illness of both substance and spirit. Taking half-measures or shirking the full responsibility for one's personal transformation would not do.

If illness and healing are to become meaningful processes in our lives, the transformative experience must be sought after and fully accepted. It is only through the process of transformation that pain is forced to reveal its *meaning*. Humanity suffers illness, but it also has the propensity to *transcend* suffering. Whitmont says that illness "brings to the fore an implicate archetype that wants to incarnate and be woven into the web of life."

If we refuse this challenge, the hero's "call to adventure," to participate fully in our own development—our becoming of who we are meant to be—we not only fail to be healed, but we cannot be saved. Though we might be "cured" by bypass surgery or some such medical intervention, the "broken heart," though "fixed," won't be made truly whole again. Only acceptance of the necessary process of transformation and *cooperation with it* can achieve that.

chapter four
The Healing Journey

Healing seems to be a function of restoring or reweaving the torn fabric of life in some way. The vital factors in the healing process...include intention, motivation, trust, and something as ineffable as passion for living. When suffering and tragedy are transformed and colored with meaning and purpose, healing has surely occurred, by whatever means, and under whatever circumstances.

～ Jeanne Achterberg, Ph.D.
Rituals of Healing

~ *Healing Mind, Body, Spirit*

All healing is a journey, and every journey contains the seeds of transformation. The hope of tomorrow is planted in the seeds of today. Whether we allow them to sprout and then water and tend them to the fulfillment of bloom is up to us. Just as a seed contains within it the pattern of the whole plant—root, shoot, stem, leaf, bud, flower, fruit—we contain within ourselves the blueprint for what we are capable of becoming.

When we travel, either physically or mentally, we open ourselves to new and transformative experiences—*or not*. An unforgettable incident that befell me at the Lisbon airport illustrates this point.

The last leg of a year in Europe had been a month in Portugal, on a *finca* (farm) in the Algarve, miles from "civilization," with no public electricity in the area. Donkey carts were the farmers' primary mode of transportation. A private generator at the *finca* supplied electric power three hours each day. My traveling companion had to accustom himself to a single midday shave; I cooked the day's food in one session. A small ice-chest provided minimal refrigeration; potable water came out of huge bottles.

In the absolute absence of artificial light, I experienced for the first time the kind of dark one only hears about—where you cannot see your hand in front of your face. So thick was the dark that at night, we dared not venture a foot out of doors without a flashlight. The sky, thick with stars as a field with daisies, appeared as the ancients must have seen it. "Diamonds on black velvet" is an apt description. Its star-strewn magnificence was awe-inspiring.

Every hour stretched my mind and senses, expanding my horizons and changing my perspectives. Beauty abounded. Walking in the orange grove at the foot of our villa, where hundreds of globes of lucent color hung among the glossy green leaves, was more like being in a fragrant painting than in a garden. A tall hedge of mimosa stretching as far as the eye could see softly perfumed the air, its golden bloom adding to the artist's palette of a myriad of wildflowers.

The almond trees—those first heralds of spring—were in bloom, their snowy blossoms on leafless branches looking like white cotton candy. Patient farmers with handplows worked centuries-old terraced hillsides just as their ancestors had done. In between orchards, the sun-drenched hills were covered with flowering plants in brilliant colors of magenta, yellow, purple, red.

So many rich experiences: shopping at the bustling open-air market; discovering exquisite tiled alleyways while wandering lost; buying fish and unknown sea creatures on the beach from grizzled fishermen beside their brightly colored boats; wandering long stretches of empty white sand and exploring rock caves beside the sparkling blue ocean. At night we were stirred by the lilting soft-toned sounds of *fado*, the bittersweet love songs of Portugal. Sometimes I wept into my wine.

During my wondrous time in Portugal, I met with nothing but kindness and courtesy from a gentle people, who, though poor, are steeped in the milk of human kindness. Though my companion and I spoke only about five words of Portuguese, *obrigado* (thank you) and a few hand signals took us everywhere we wanted to go and provided all the necessary communications. It was a sad day for me when I had to leave and return to my life in New York. At the Lisbon airport I parted from my friend, who was returning to Holland, and, heavy-hearted to leave a land that had given me so much to treasure, waited for my flight to be called.

Because I was traveling with my cat, I was preboarded onto the minibus that took passengers to the airplane. I sat alone in silence on the little conveyance, gazing fondly and forlornly at the hills beyond the tarmac, lost in a welter of abundant memories, new perceptions, and feelings. A few months earlier I had suffered a bout of depression from a sense of futility about my life. Now I was renewed: I felt reborn into a new harmony.

Suddenly, there stormed aboard the miniscule bus a raucous American tourist group, wearing bright shorts, straw hats, and fresh sunburns. Festooned with cameras and carrying cheap, plastic tote bags stuffed with the souvenirs every country provides for tourists, they shrieked in ear-splitting merriment their elation at returning to "the good old U.S.A." where everyone spoke English and where there were elevators and plenty of electricity. Insensitive to the presence of a Portuguese driver and hostess, they loudly disparaged everything about the country whose hospitality they had recently enjoyed: the people, the land, the language, the food, their accommodations, the lack of "civilized" amenities and comforts.

The loud leader of the pack stood over me. I looked up at his sunburned face, into his bright blue eyes, and said, "If you like the States so much, why didn't you *stay* there?"

Though I had spoken quietly, my vehemence was felt. A ripple of ashamed silence pulsed through the group, subduing them.

Unless you open yourself to the *adventure* life offers, your journey will have been in vain. You can suffer illness or pain and take nothing from the experience except the memory of your suffering and perhaps resentment and anger at the vicissitudes of life. In *The Symbolic Quest*, Whitmont says,

> While suffering thus remains suffering, a legitimate part of experience, it may become more bearable if it is seen as a road that can lead not only to pain and annihilation but also to a widening and deepening of one's sense of being. Illness attains a higher dignity once it is recognized not only as senseless wastefulness but also as meaningful experience.

The Healing Journey

~ Illness as Mask

Illness serves many purposes for different people. At its peak, it can be a means of self-transformation that takes us to a higher spiritual level. At its nadir, it can be the route of escape from life. It can be a screen behind which we hide our true feelings and desires, from others or from ourselves. It can also be used to refuse true maturity, to manipulate or control others, or as a means of coping with difficulties.

For example, a wife and mother of three, approaching "empty nest syndrome," wanted a new baby to fill the gaping void. Her husband instead had his heart set on quitting his high-paying but unfulfilling job to go out on his own as a consultant. She feared this move and the financial insecurity it would bring. Knowing he would veto having another child, she secretly discontinued her birth control.

Not surprisingly, a pregnancy resulted from this deception and, being a responsible man, he had no choice but to accept this wrench thrust into the spokes of his own ambition. With college tuition for three boys already staring him in the face, his hope of a solo career was smashed and he was now fettered to his job for life.

He concealed his anger and disappointment, outwardly accepting the coming "happy event," but his unspoken resentment simmered like a stew in a kettle. The pregnancy was a time of acute tension between them. As if in response to the unspoken conflict between her parents, the child was born covered with an eczema-type rash and had to be hospitalized several times in infancy.

The husband's previously unflagging romantic ardor for his wife cooled. He stopped approaching her for sex and spoke no words of love. She felt him slipping away from her. Within a year of the birth, she became mysteriously ill. First one vague symptom bothered her, and then another. Fevers, skin rashes, internal pain plagued her.

For two years she was intermittently hospitalized. Her worried husband became fearful of losing the mother of his children. Though she had every organ biopsied, her complaints remained mystifying to a host of specialists, and as the bills mounted, the husband was even more locked into his job. Each time she was hospitalized for yet another test, it increased the load of anxiety he carried, and each time he became more and more attentive, lovingly expressing his concern and hope for her complete recovery.

No diagnosis was ever made. Loving sexual relations resumed. The child became "Daddy's little girl." There was no more talk of him quitting his job. Having served its purpose, the mysterious ailment vanished as curiously as it had appeared, and she recovered her health completely.

The relatively helpless state of illness can be used to disguise one's psychological dependency needs, by getting them met covertly. An example is the case of a man brought down by the loss of his job. As long as he was the breadwinner, he could demand that him wife stay home and take care of him. Bereft of his breadwinner status, with the props underneath his macho stance knocked out, this man was suddenly no longer in a position to require his wife's total attention. In fact, she had to go out and get a job herself in order to help support them.

Morose, he moped about the house, growing ever more dependent emotionally and getting less and less attention. Holding down a job, meantime, was making his wife more independent and self-assertive, and when she suggested that he get a job—any job—to tide them over, even if it meant working below his previous salary and skills, he promptly fell ill. His blood pressure shot up dangerously. He had heart palpitations. The doctor said, "stress," and recommended complete rest.

Now, he had his wife's full attention, even though she continued to work. No more demands were made for him to take a job beneath his capabilities.

Fortunately for this man, his doctor—realizing there was more to the situation than met the medical eye—recommended psychotherapy. He learned about his unacknowledged dependency needs, learned that it was OK to have needs, learned that he was responsible for fulfilling his own needs. Couples' counseling ensued and both spouses were made aware of the hidden dynamics of their relationship. They accepted the transformation process as being both necessary and health-giving. With time on his hands, he began to do things around the house that previously he had depended on his wife to do. He learned to cook and found he enjoyed it, happily surprising his wife with delicious gourmet dinners when she returned from her work. One thing led to another, and the two decided to combine his newly found love of cooking with her newly acquired business skills and open a small catering business, which is now thriving. His blood pressure is normal, and there is a wonderful spring in his step. When people congratulate him on his "executive comeback," he defers to his wife's considerable ability, saying with pride, "I cook the food. *She* cooks the books!"

As a place of safety as well as of learning, school for me was both respite and refuge. Any absence was fraught with danger. Every year at the Christmas season, I came down with a severe flu that kept me secluded in my room for the full two weeks of school holiday. Though I was miserably sick, I welcomed these bouts for the protection they afforded me—prolonged contact with my father always had disastrous consequences. This syndrome, called "secondary gains," is not uncommon—it shows how illness can be used as a coping mechanism. In this context, Whitmont says, "Illness is the 'invasion' of a dynamic that arises out of the Self-field and leads to a dramatic conflict which encodes itself psychosomatically."

It is the choice we make that determines the course of the healing. We can choose, like the tourists, to take nothing from the experience of our journey, or we can choose to realize that there is important information to be gained, which can change our lives positively.

Illness and the Shadow

In Jungian terms, the "shadow" is the repressed or unrealized part of the personality, which goes underground and causes no end of trouble. The shadow is that element in us that we are least willing to admit is a part of us. It consists of personal qualities that constitute the part of ourselves we consider "dark," or unacceptable, and therefore reject or refuse to acknowledge. Though we cannot see our shadows, others have no trouble observing the contradiction between how we perceive ourselves and how we really are. Inside the altruistic do-gooder may reside a hidden egoist with selfish intent; the man of courage may harbor a coward; the sweetest of sweethearts, a jealous vixen. Often projected onto another person—in the "It's not me, it's *him*" syndrome—the shadow can also be projected *through* illness, allowing the person to use the illness as a vehicle for objectifying the shadow.

An example of this is the woman who regards herself as the epitome of loving concern for others. Her perception of herself is that she is *always* doing good deeds; *always* putting her own needs last, *always* there when others need her, especially her family.

She views herself as a "giving" person, with no ulterior motives behind her altruism, but her shadow side desperately wants and needs the attention she gives to others—purportedly to fulfill *their* needs. The shadow side of her vaunted altruism is an immature neediness, which, denying, she projects onto others, claiming they need *her* help.

In return for her giving, she expects to be given to—all the time, upon demand—and to have her needs anticipated by those around her, for whom she has cared so dearly. Because she doesn't acknowledge her craving, thinking it wrong, she demands attention covertly, often getting ill as a means to this end. She projects this "shadow" *through* her illness, a device that allows it to play itself out without disturbing her picture of herself as a totally giving, unselfish, undemanding, loving person. "Look at all I have done for you," is her aggrieved attitude toward others, who, in time, find her demands intolerable and avoid her company. Unfortunately, this only serves to reinforce her concept of herself as a martyr.

The way out of the impasse is to "own" the shadow. When we acknowledge that we are projecting qualities in ourselves, we neutralize the shadow's ability to do harm. The woman in the previous example uses her "weakness" as a shield against acknowledging the ruthless tyrant within who wants to dominate everyone, but doesn't dare do this openly. Recognizing the shadow self and acknowledging its legitimate role enables us to become more fully our SELF. "When there is an impasse [illness]...we must look to the dark, hitherto unacceptable side which has not been at our conscious disposal, and that the shadow, when realized, is the source of renewal," says Whitmont.

~ The Wounded Healer

A disproportionate number of people who are either physically or emotionally wounded choose "helping" professions, such as health care and psychotherapy. But in order to be effective, the healer of others must not only possess certain skills but must also maintain a high degree of self-awareness and be finely tuned to his or her own ongoing inner processes. It is well known that a kind of symbiotic energy draws patients or clients to certain doctors or therapists. Freud's patients tended to prove his male-dominant "penis envy" theories, while the more feminine-oriented Jung was visited predominantly by women, who were receptive to his methods and point of view. The practitioner must therefore be very clear about what wounds or has wounded him or her.

For the person seeking to be his or her own healer, the process is essentially the same. How does the wounded person become a "wounded healer," or a wounded *self-healer*? By achieving and maintaining a high degree of awareness, by accepting the inevitable state of woundedness as part of the condition of being alive, and by seeking inwardly for the *meaning* of wounds received or self-inflicted. When this woundedness is assimilated and accepted, it radiates out great healing power directly into the psychic and biologic bloodstream of the individual. As a by-product, it also creates a "healing personality" that enables each one of us to become a wounded healer for others in some way.

Before I became a therapist, a dear friend, who had suffered a breakdown in the wake of a bitter divorce and subsequently had to resign from a job he loved, asked me to accompany him on a trip to the wilds of Maine, his original home. We took an isolated cabin near the water and spent our time without entertainment or social activity.

It was a brooding place, bleak and stark—a reflection of his state of mind and being. We walked by the water's edge, stood on rocky promontories and let the cold seaspray soak us, bought lobsters off a fishing boat, picnicked on the deserted beach, and were silent a lot of the time. At night, we ate simple dinners I cooked in the rustic cabin, drank wine, and went early to sleep. At the end of the trip, as we were at the airport in Portland waiting for our flight back to New York City, he suddenly grasped my hand warmly and exclaimed, "Thank you *so much*. You've saved my life."

Astonished at this declaration, for I had done nothing unusual and had in fact thoroughly enjoyed myself, I said, "You're welcome, but I didn't *do* anything."

My puzzlement must have communicated itself to him strongly, for he squeezed my hand tightly and said, by way of explanation, "You didn't need to do anything. You have a healing personality."

I never forgot that statement. He subsequently returned to his full powers, but it was more than twenty years later that I read, in Whitmont's *The Alchemy of Healing*, "The doctor's very personality is a potent influence upon the patient and the therapeutic process."

To become wounded healers to ourselves or to others, we must use the death of the restricting and limiting past as the *prima materia* and "cook" it in the crucible of our trauma. We must accept and honor our wounds as sacred vessels in which we transmute our pain into the "uncommon gold" of self-realization. Then, with poet Howard Moss, we can declare, "My wound has been my healing and I am made more beautiful by losses."

Traveler's Aid: Flower Essences

Emotions can kill you. Emotional harmony and balance are the basis of health and well-being. Negative thoughts are as dangerous to your health as bacteria and viruses. Positive thoughts and feelings can even protect you from becoming infected. And, if you do become ill or have an accident, the power of a positive outlook will speed your natural healing process.

Flower essences are described for emotional or psychological conditions or types, but they often result in improvements on the physical level as well. Because they penetrate to the implicate order through subtle vibrational means, as do homeopathic preparations used to treat physical problems, they can be extraordinarily effective over a broad range of conditions. My ten years of studying and using them for myself and my clients has proved them efficacious in improving health through restoring emotional balance.

Flower essence remedies are homeopathic preparations one can easily self-prescribe. Numerous books are available on the subject, as are tests that can be self-given to determine which remedies apply to you. (See Appendix Two.)

The essences come in liquid form and are administered diluted in pure water. Extracted from flowers and plants, they are not a drug or a chemical but derive from the traditional idea that plants contain healing properties. In fact, many of our drugs are based on plant derivatives or synthetic replicates of them. The ingredient in aspirin, for example, was originally extracted from the bark of the willow tree.

The theory behind essences is the same as I have already posited: that our inner states affect our physical condition. It is well known, for example, that so-called Type-A people, with a tough, aggressive, hard-driving style, are at risk for heart disease. Now it is being recognized, according to a study by psychologist Tilmer Engebretson at Ohio State University in Columbus, that people who have a trait he names "cynical hostility" are at greater risk for developing heart-tissue damage than are their nonhostile colleagues. Other reports have shown a connection between hostility in healthy people and the subsequent development of atherosclerosis and high cholesterol. One study at Duke University showed that cynicism, mistrust, and aggressive anger hiked the death rate from heart disease.

By treating these emotional stress conditions that underlie disease and illness, we get at the root of the problem directly. Real and lasting change in attitudes toward themselves and others are readily observed by those who take the remedies. It may seem odd to you that flower extracts can make such far-reaching changes to a personality, but the effectiveness of the flower essences has been demonstrated.

The oldest flower essences are the Bach Flower Remedies, developed in England in the 1930s by Dr. Edward Bach, a physician who was dismayed at the lack of success he was achieving with the medical methods of his day. He gave up a successful practice to devote himself exclusively to finding remedies in the plant world that would enable his suffering patients to overcome the emotional conditions that beset them—fear, worry, depression—and to assist in their own healing. The remedies are still prepared exclusively by the Dr. Edward Bach Healing Center in England. Of them, John Diamond, M.D., says,

> [T]here is no doubt of their tremendous efficacy. They are as potent as any therapeutic substances that we have for raising the life energy of the individual. Dr. Bach never meant them to be therapeutic in the sense of primarily curing physical disease, but rather as overcoming the mental correlates of physical disease so as to allow the inhibited life energy to manifest itself and to proceed with the healing process, the true healing—that which comes from within.

Some examples are Vine for the desire to control and dominate; Willow for resentment and bitterness; Chicory for possessive martyr types; Heather for the lonely and self-absorbed; and White Chestnut for the worried and mentally obsessing. A special blend of essences used to treat emergency conditions such as shock, whether physical or emotional, is called "Rescue Remedy." I keep a small bottle in my purse. The remedies can be placed directly under the tongue if water is not available. My diabetic cat once went into convulsions, and I saved his life by putting a drop of the Rescue Remedy on his tongue. Another especially useful remedy is Star of Bethlehem, one of the components of the Rescue Remedy. It is for the *aftereffect* of shock, whether mental or physical, and is for anyone who has suffered trauma, especially in childhood. Dr. Bach called this remedy, "The comforter and soother of pains and sorrows."

Similar to the Rescue Remedy is "Five-Flower Formula," from Healing Herbs English Flower Essences. The California Flower Essences, developed during the 1970s, reflect their era. They are specific to conditions such as spiritual growth and self-actualization, alienation and isolation—all New Age concerns. Some examples are Shooting Star for feeling alienated; Dogwood for receptivity to love; Mariposa Lily for the feeling of separateness; and Bleeding Heart for releasing painful emotional attachments.

The remedies can be used alone or as enhancements for the visualizations and affirmations in the following chapters. It is best to take no more than four at one time. Think of them as lifelong friends. Change them as *you* change, carefully selecting them for your current state. If you use a pendulum, you can check your selections with it. The essences will be a comforting companion on your healing journey.

chapter five
Advice to the Traveler

Most of what we ascribe to random or accidental behavior is actually an expression of an unconscious, creative depth-awareness which expresses a goal-directed activity of an evolving transpersonal dynamic that both includes and transcends personal rational functioning.

Edward C. Whitmont, M.D.
The Alchemy of Healing

When one goes on a journey into unfamiliar territory, it is best to have a knowledgeable guide who knows the terrain, speaks the language, and is familiar with the customs. Wise and serious travelers also keep journals to record experiences and impressions of the new territory being explored and to compare it to what already has been seen. Consciousness of individual temperament, or type, allows for advance planning so that the conditions are provided that will make the trip a success.

Your Healing Guide

A guide is actually a symbol for our own deepest wisdom, which resides in the SELF and connects us to all the other SELF-entities everywhere, to nonhuman life, to nonorganic life, to the cosmos itself.

During my life, I have encountered many guides. You, too, will have more than one guide during your lifetime, but you can call upon cosmic tour guides at any time you feel you need guidance.

A guide may present itself as an "archetype"—an old man or a wise woman; a human figure you may or may not recognize, such as a grandparent or an idealized teacher; an animal that talks or communicates telepathically; a spiritual entity, such as an angel or "intelligence" from another dimension; or even as a rock or body of water. These symbols are likely to shift and change over time and with the subject for which you are asking guidance. Asking for guidance with healing may produce a figure consonant with your idea of a healer. Accept what comes, for it arises from your deepest SELF.

By making the effort to meet and dialogue with your healing guide, you will be setting a precedent for getting help on a regular, sometimes unasked-for basis. Your healing guide can warn you of incipient problems in advance of real illness; it can provide you with penetrating insight into what ails you; it can reveal subtle nuances of meaning that are embedded in your experience of illness and healing.

For example, one man contacted a guide whom he saw as a long-bearded, gray-haired old man of great age. He called him "Methuselah" after the biblical figure and felt great comfort in the presence of this ancient one who seemed to be all-knowing. He enjoyed making this contact and relished the sense of trust he felt with this guide.

Once, he developed a series of painful migraine headaches for which his doctor made no other than the usual "stress" diagnosis. Unsatisfied and often in crippling pain, he contacted Methuselah and asked him what the trouble was. That night in a dream, he saw the old man coming out of an operating room holding in his hand what looked like a Ping-Pong ball. He tossed this object to the man, who caught it, noticing that it seemed filled with fluid.

Intrigued by this image, the man called his doctor and asked for a CAT scan but was told it was not necessary. As his HMO would not pay for any unauthorized tests, he let the matter go. A few days later, he was hit by one of the unexplained migraine headaches, which doubled him over with pain. That night, sedated as he was, he "saw" a vision of the old man in sorrowful mien standing over his unconscious body. At first he thought the vision was the product of the drugs he had been given for the intense pain, but then he got a strong feeling that his guide was showing him a future possibility. Alarmed, he decided to demand the CAT scan, even if he had to foot the bill himself. He got the test, which revealed a small fluid-filled cyst on his brain. It was benign and easily removed; after the healing process the man had no more headaches.

Much relieved, and thankful, he did a meditation to tell Methuselah that all had gone well and to ask him to monitor his brain in the future. To his utter surprise, the old man admonished him severely, saying sternly, "You have missed the point." What point? The cyst was removed, all was well—what could the remark mean?

The man meditated on the image of the Ping-Pong ball, seeing it flying through the air, back and forth, back and forth. Slowly, it dawned on him that this was how he lived his life. He'd been taught at business school to "Keep your eye on the ball," and that's all he had ever done, becoming a workaholic. But Ping-Pong was a *game*—it was supposed to be *fun*. The "game of life" was supposed to be fun, too, but it had turned into a fiercely competitive sport in which winning was the only acceptable outcome. Realizing that the cyst represented a deeper imbalance than a mere physical disorder, he vowed to change his ways.

Meeting Your Guide

In this meditation, you are going to meet a healing guide whom you can trust and rely on. To prepare yourself, do the following:

1. Articulate a question you wish to ask your guide. State the question as clearly and succinctly as you can. Vague questions beget vague answers. The more specific the question, the more specific the answer will be.
2. Choose a question that cannot be answered by a simple *yes* or *no*. The purpose of the first effort to contact a guide is for you to get to know this realm of your inside being.
3. Stick to your present situation and avoid broad generalities. Don't ask, "How can I get well?" or "What's the matter with me?" Instead, phrase a question specifically, as in "My upper right arm is stiff and painful. What can you advise me about this condition?"

Advice to the Traveler

4. Choose a question that does not require a prediction. This is usually interpreted as trying to "test" the guide. Simply asking for guidance is always good. State the subject about which you wish guidance.
5. Be willing to trust your guide and to accept whatever form will appear to you.
6. Remind yourself to pay attention to the guide's appearance. You will ask your guide for a name or a symbol by which you can recognize him or her in the future.

After you have prepared yourself for your encounter with your guide, find the time to be alone and undisturbed for half an hour. Relax yourself completely and let go of the day's tensions and cares.

Mentally take yourself to a place somewhere in nature—a forest, the seaside, a flower-filled meadow, a lake shore, a cove—whatever appeals to you. See in front of you in this pleasant place a veiled object, full of mystery. A puff of wind comes along and blows away the covering, and your guide is revealed to you. Take whatever image comes and begin to dialogue with it. Ask your question and wait for an answer. If one doesn't come immediately, be patient. The answer may come in words, through intuition or telepathy, as an image, or even as a snatch of song or an instruction to read a book or magazine article.

In these guided meditations, the specifics are not as important as making the contact. Whatever springs into your mind is the right answer, because you are using a process to contact your own inner wisdom. Your guides are within the realm of the deepest part of your being, which is connected to all reality everywhere at all times and places.

When you have met your guide, introduced yourself, and asked your question, notice the details of the place so that you can return here whenever you like. Fix it in your memory. When you get the answer to your question, thank your guide and say you will look forward to further dialogue in the future.

If you do not get an answer, or if the answer seems to make no sense, accept that also and try again later. Remember, you are learning a new skill.

If you are asking about pain or illness, ask your guide what your pain is trying to tell you. Ask what its deeper meaning is.

Before leaving, make an appointment to meet with your guide again at a set time. Follow through on this with another meditation.

~ Keeping a Healing Journal

All travelers are advised to keep a record of their journey. A healing journal is an adjunct to your regular healing practice and will serve as a channel into your own intuition about yourself and your health.

Record your thoughts and feelings along with physical circumstances. Jot down which meditations you use, and what results are obtained.

In time, you will perceive patterns of meaning. Your life is not an accidental or random event; it has meaning and purpose. Keeping a healing journal will help you to discover this.

If you are already a journal-keeper, this will be no problem. If you are new to journal-keeping, you may need some time to acclimate yourself to writing about your healing experiences on a regular basis. Whatever you do, make it an *enjoyable* experience. Play with the journal. You don't have to restrict yourself to writing in words; you can draw or paste pictures in it, or copy healing affirmations or bits of poetry. One friend makes it a habit to write down a self-created affirmation, a sort of ode to her healing process, each day.

Use any form you please. I find a bound notebook is best because I tend to lose separate pieces of paper. A simple spiral notebook is inexpensive and widely available, or you may prefer something grander, such as a cloth-bound book with blank pages.

Rereading what you have written, whether the next day or a year later, can be an illuminating experience. For one thing, you may be little aware of your progress until you see where you were this time last year. *Enjoy* your journal—think of it as a dear friend with whom you spend intimate time.

How much time you spend with your healing journal is up to you. During a six-month period when I was undergoing an intense healing after a plunge into the pit of depression, I wrote many pages every day. In fact, keeping my healing journal became, for that period of time, my life work. Many of those experiences are reflected here. Had I not written it all down, I might have forgotten many of the lessons I learned, lost the details of my healing journey, or even had the whole experience fade away like last summer's flowers.

Write when and for how long or how much it suits you each time. If you are a person who responds well to a scheduled activity, by all means put it in your schedule. If not—and I think this is preferable—let it be spontaneous. Whatever works for you at the time is best.

Of course, if you are going through a specific illness, such as a surgical procedure, you may have a lot of time for reflection and writing during your recuperation period. Don't waste it watching reruns on TV. You will find much more interesting material inside yourself.

In addition to keeping your journal on a regular basis, you can benefit by writing out your *feelings* about any particularly traumatic experience. This technique was developed by James W. Pennebaker, Ph.D., a professor in the psychology department of Southern Methodist University. To do this technique, spend twenty minutes writing about the most traumatic experience relating to your health condition. Write nonstop and don't be concerned about spelling or grammar.

Often, emotions will pour forth, even tears—but these are healing tears of release. This is an excellent method to gain insight into the meaning of your illness or pain; such insights help you cope with the stress involved in any illness or discomfort. Patients report that the writing exercise served to improve their emotional and physical well-being on a long-term basis.

When doing this technique, it is important to continue it for at least four days in a row, or longer. The reason is that writing out feelings about deeply wounding experiences just once will only reopen the wound but not suffice to begin healing it. According to Pennebaker, the patients who wrote about their deepest feelings related to trauma experienced remarkable benefits in both physical and emotional health, compared to control groups who wrote only about trivial events. The immune systems of the first group were strengthened, leading Pennebaker to conclude that expressing emotions can enhance physical health. He says, "Just putting upsetting experiences into words has profound psychological and physical benefits for our participants."

His reasoning is that repressing feelings is a *physiological* strain—blood pressure, heart rate, muscle tension all increase when emotions are "stuffed," or blocked from being expressed. Pennebaker theorizes that when we express our long-buried emotions in words, we relieve the body as well as the mind of crippling stress. His studies have proved that the expression of thoughts and feelings can affect our overall health positively. He suggests the journal method be used to heal past traumas, as well as to relieve ongoing present-day stresses.

The Bach Flower Remedy *Star of Bethlehem*, for neutralizing the shocks to the system that manifest in the body as illness, is an excellent adjunct to this process. Another good choice is *Walnut*, for breaking the links with the past, especially recommended for those who have suffered early trauma of any kind and can't seem to get free of its effects. The Remedy *White Chestnut* is suggested for those who are plagued by constant thoughts of some distressing experience, leaving them both mentally and physically exhausted.

Your healing journal can also be a way to help yourself lessen stress and handle anxiety or depression. Whatever your goal, making a commitment to writing on a regular basis is the key to success.

Discovering Your Healing Type

Your healing type is imprinted at the moment of birth by the elemental distribution of your inborn nature. Harmonizing with your personal element makeup is an excellent way both to prevent illness and to augment or restore health. The elements represent our "personal weather," both emotionally and physically.

How we respond to the challenge illness presents is of utmost importance to the healing process. Focusing on your healing type will help you to restore your body to health or prevent sickness from occurring. Your type reveals much about your natural tendencies toward ill health and your attitude toward your healing process.

A major factor, also influenced by type, is one's self-image and general attitude toward one's life. These fundamentally influence our constitutional and immune system reactions on the physical plane. And because they are susceptible to being changed, we possess much more healing power than we know.

◁─▷ *Healing Mind, Body, Spirit*

By mobilizing our transformative abilities through the use of the various tools and techniques now available to us, we can reach deep into the implicate order and effect far-reaching change, which will in turn spread through the total organism.

There are four basic types, related to Fire, Earth, Water, and Air. You may be a single type, a mixture of two types, or a multiple type. Also, you may find emphasis on one type or another (especially if you are a mixed type) at different times of the month, day, year, or over a lifespan.

You must determine your natural affinity for each of the four elements. From this information, you will derive your type. Then, tune in to your basic type and learn to work with its healing energy.

You are now going to discover your healing type. Treat this exercise like a game—consider it an exploration of the unknown territory of your enfolded SELF.

From the word lists that follow, choose *only* the words that apply to you. Make four columns that rate the degree to which each word applies: *always, often, rarely,* or *never*. The idea is for you to make contact with your deep inner SELF's implicate order, or innate elemental pattern.

Let the process flow from your interior self until you feel you have finished. Choose as many or as few words as you like. You don't have to work in any particular order—go back and forth between the lists if you like.

One way to approach this is to first read a list quickly and then spontaneously choose words that produce a strong emotional charge, either positive—*Yes! Always!*—or negative—*No! Never!* After that, go back and choose those that fall into the "often" or "rarely" categories.

Advice to the Traveler

~ The Four Types

Fire

Self-starting	Self-aware	Blunt
Self-confident	Dramatic	Outdoors-
Action-initiating	Playful	oriented
Decisive	Fun-loving	Travel-oriented
Outgoing	Powerful	Careless
Forceful	Impressive	Explosive
Driving	Enthusiastic	Foolhardy
Active	Expansive	Egotistical
Strong	Optimistic	Jovial
Adventurous	Generous	Proud
Self-expressive	Outgoing	Willful

Earth

Organized	Detail-oriented	Deliberate
Serious	Methodical	Money-oriented
Practical	Sensible	Prudent
Down-to-earth	Businesslike	Cautious
Realistic	Sanitary	Economical
Ambitious	Stable	Self-controlled
Hardworking	Steady	Reserved
Structured	Reliable	Pessimistic
Methodical	Productive	Factual
Disciplined	Persistent	Helpful
Analytical	Determined	Dutiful

Air

Communicative	Sociable	Original
Quick-witted	Companionable	Individualistic
Inquisitive	Just	Nonconformist
Adaptable	Balanced	Charming
Curious	Tolerant	Refined
Versatile	Impartial	Studious
Flexible	Intellectually	Babbling
Variety-seeking	detached	Nervous
Relationship-	Friendly	Superficial
oriented	Innovative	Mentally
Cooperative	Independent	organized

Water

Feeling	Passionate	Artistic
Sensitive	Secretive	Inspired
Sympathetic	Mysterious	Receptive
Nostalgic	Compassionate	Moody
Comfort-loving	Benevolent	Clinging
Security-oriented	Sentimental	Brooding
Domestic	Intuitive	Emotionally
Family-oriented	Escapist	perceptive
Food-oriented	Spacey	Passive
Emotional	Impractical	Instinctive
Intense	Unrealistic	Spiritual

If you choose *only* words from a single list, then you are a pure type (this is rare). Most people will have at least a few words from at least two elemental categories. To determine your type, first count the words *from each list* that you have placed

Advice to the Traveler

into each column. The highest number of words from any one list in your "always" column determines your primary type.

For example, if you chose twenty words from the "Fire" category and placed them in the "always" column but chose fewer than twenty words from any or all of the other categories for this column, then you are a basic Fire Type. Having determined your primary type, next count the words in your "often" column. If the highest number of these words comes from the *same* element as those in your "always" column, then more emphasis is placed upon the primary type.

If, however, an equal or greater number of words comes from a *different* list, you have a secondary type. For example, if you are a basic Fire Type but the highest number of words in the "often" category is from the Water list, you are a mixed Fire-Water type.

The next step is to determine if you have a missing or inferior (de-emphasized) element. To do this, follow the same procedure outlined above and check the "never" category, which will indicate a missing element. Then check the "rarely" category, which will indicate an inferior element.

A missing or de-emphasized element means that there is an imbalance; ideally, all four elements would be represented. When this occurs (and it is common), you can "add" the missing element by consciously seeking to tune in to it. For example, if Earth is missing, then you can add earth-grounding by planting a garden, working with the hands, or just sitting on the ground and tuning in to Mother Nature. Similarly, you can add Water by going to the seaside or lakeshore, taking long soaks in the tub, or walking in the rain.

Sometimes, we get elementally out of balance. This might be the case when a Water Type is forced to go on a family camping trip in the mountains, or, conversely, when an Air Type has to spend time in the moist air of a lakeside or beside the ocean. When the stress of ordinary living causes an imbalance to occur, illness can follow. Your elemental balance provides important clues to the maintenance of health and the means of healing. Allowing ourselves to be "in our element" is a wonderful curative.

The "Pure" Types

The Fire Type

The energy of Fire is radiant. Your energy is flowing and you are excitable, enthusiastic, impatient, spontaneous, quick to react, self-centered, and overly objective. Your natural high spirits give you self-esteem. Strength comes in spurts. A strong desire for self-expression and the need for freedom are your dominant characteristics.

Being cooped up depletes your life force; you need vigorous physical activity during the daytime, preferably out in the sunshine, with as much contact with the sun as possible. Winter in cold climates is hard on you, but sufficient outdoor activity during the hot summer months will allow you to store your elemental energy against the gloom of indoor winter months. Your energy goes down when the sun does. Early to bed, early to rise is a good health habit.

Illness, which can be brought on by overexcitement and a lack of proper rest, is difficult for you as you dislike being confined and inactive. You need to develop patience with illness or infirmity; premature return to activity can bring on a relapse. Restore balance by incorporating sunlight into your healing process. You are prone to the syndrome known as SAD, or seasonal affective disorder, caused by lack of sunlight. Light treatment can help.

You tend to suffer from headaches; injuries resulting from impulsive behavior; heart problems due to overwork and overactivity; and chronic back pain, which is often the product of lack of rest.

When you are ill or recovering, other Fire Types are healing for you because they replenish your energy. Air Types are good, but they can tire you with their endless mental speculations. Avoid Earth and Water Types: Earth smothers you; Water drenches your Fire.

Some flower remedies that will help to renew you are Heather, for self-centeredness; Impatiens, for lack of patience; Hornbeam, for mental and physical exhaustion; and Vervain, for tension and stress.

The Earth Type

The energy of Earth is related closely to the physical plane and senses. Your energy is stable and you are patient, reliable, hardworking, commonsensical, practical, and stubborn. You have extraordinary stamina. The desire for concrete results and the self-discipline needed to get them are your dominant characteristics.

You need to be in physical contact with your element. You need to get your hands and feet into the soil, and to handle growing things and the solid basic material of the Earth, such as rocks and minerals. Crystal therapy often works wonders for Earth Types.

Though you have great physical stamina, you are not inclined to physical exertion, and you need to push yourself to exercise regularly. You need to go at your own pace, especially in the matter of sleeping and waking. Being rushed can make you ill, literally, or delay recovery. When ill, you recuperate slowly, but steadily and thoroughly. Pragmatic even when ill, you are a serene patient *if* you are convinced the treatment will produce concrete results.

You tend to have throat problems, to get colds with sore throats as a result of emotional congestion or pushing your endurance level beyond its limit by continuing to work long past time to rest. You are prone to digestive upsets resulting from nerves and your desire for perfection. Bones can be brittle—women especially need to guard against osteoporosis—and teeth can cause problems. Regular dental checkups are a must. Skin, too, is sensitive and can become dry and scaly if not cared for properly. Restore balance by cultivating your sensuous side, not only when ill but as a preventative measure. Massage and scented body lotions are good choices.

When ill or recovering, associating with Fire people energizes you, and you find Water Types soothing. Other Earth Types can make the atmosphere too heavy; avoid Air Types, whose lack of common sense annoys you.

Some flower remedies that will help to renew you are Beech, to combat self-criticism; Chicory, for possessiveness; Mustard, for melancholy; and Oak, for heavy responsibilities.

The Air Type

The energy of Air is ephemeral. Your energy is constantly shifting, and you are mental, abstract, detached, fair-minded, talkative, diplomatic, and multifaceted. Detaching from the "messy" human emotions and emphasizing theory and concepts are your dominant characteristics.

Prolonged contact with wet air depletes you, and in a humid climate, you should have a dehumidifier in your room. You find emotional display upsetting; an atmosphere heavy with emotion can make you ill. Witnessing or coping with outbursts of weeping or temperament can bring on exhaustion. You prefer to talk about emotions rationally rather than actually dealing with them, but repressing your own emotions can cause illness.

You have nervous energy and need to dissipate it with mental activity in order to get a good night's sleep, but allow sufficient time to wind down before bed, which is a good time to spend a quiet half hour in meditation. It's important for you to maintain a calm restful environment to counteract your inclination to live in your busy head.

When ill, you want to know everything about what ails you. You research your diagnosis extensively, talking to everyone involved in your health care. Though you hate being confined to bed, you can deal with it if you have plenty of mental stimulation in a calm, unemotional atmosphere. Restore balance by frequent breathing exercises.

You are susceptible to respiratory ailments, especially those affecting the lungs, such as pneumonia. You are likely to dislocate a shoulder, injure your arms and hands (carpal tunnel syndrome is a risk), suffer a broken hip, or sprain an ankle. Kidney problems and circulation difficulties can arise.

When you are ill or recovering, fellow Air Types provide the mental stimulation and empathy you need; Fire Types are energizing. Avoid Earth Types, since you find their practicality depressing, and Water Types, whose emotionality gets on your nerves.

Some flower remedies that will help to renew you are Agrimony, for worry underneath the cheerfulness; Olive, for mental fatigue; White Chestnut, for persistent mental arguments and conversations; and Wild Oat, for indecision and for endlessly reviewing options.

The Water Type

The energy of Water is flowing. You are sensitive, intuitive, emotional, psychic, imaginative, and insecure. Various intangibles play a large part in your life. Being exquisitely tuned in to feelings—your own and other people's—and being very aware of your unconscious processes, which you access through dreams and intuition, are your dominant characteristics.

Although your feeling responses can go from extreme compassion to total self-pity, you trust your inner promptings and act on them. When your feelings are blocked or repressed, you can suffer psychosomatic ailments. You need to express feelings freely, for if they stay inside, they solidify into resentment and a bad temper, which can bring on ill health. When upset, you can restore balance by lying in a warm bath until feelings have settled.

Your inner landscape is forever in flux, like the ocean tides. Waves of feeling wash over you constantly; if they are not expressed, trouble results. Do not accept criticism for being "irrational," "emotional," or "overly sensitive." Insisting on the right to express feelings in a nonjudgmental atmosphere will allow you to maintain your inner harmony and physical health. You need time and space to yourself. Privacy and frequent isolation in which to sort out your complicated feelings can help you deal with stress.

When ill, you need a quiet, calm atmosphere and plenty of sleep, to promote dreaming. You respond to a spiritual environment. Meditation and prayer come easily and are of utmost importance in your healing process, which can be accelerated by soft music, preferably strings, and being near water—an ocean or a lake. Hot springs are also good. Many of your complaints are vague in nature and respond to a total-body immersion.

You can suffer immune system disorders, breast lumps, fluid retention, constipation, reproductive-system complaints, foot problems, and glandular imbalance. When ill or recovering, you benefit from the practical nature of Earth Types; other Water Types are sympathetic but feed your self-pity. Avoid Fire Types, who boil the Water nature, and Air Types, who lack empathy.

Some flower remedies that will help to renew you are Clematis, for excessive dreaminess; Honeysuckle, for overcoming nostalgic obsession; Mimulus, for fear and anxiety; and Walnut, for oversensitivity to the influence of others.

The Mixed Types

Fire/Earth

You mix practicality with impracticality, impulsiveness with patience. You can be the most reliable of persons—who suddenly goes off without notice. You can make the visionary real. You mix strength and courage. Trouble results when you are insensitive to your environment, become self-centered to the point of hypochondria, or fail to take proper health measures or precautions.

Fire/Air

You put ideas into action, join vision to logic. You are objective but can be affectionate as well. You like to gain knowledge about your own health and will seek out appropriate treatment from an intellectual standpoint. Trouble results when you disconnect from your spiritual needs and concentrate too narrowly on the intellectual level, or when you exhaust yourself through restlessness and unrealistic adventures.

Fire/Water

You are the most intuitive of the Mixed Types. You're very fluid and your connection to your inner realm is amazing. You get accurate hunches about what's wrong with you if you feel ill. Impressionable and sensitive, you respond well to visualizations to promote health and healing. Trouble results when you succumb to hysteria and overemotionalism or wall yourself off in your own private universe.

Earth/Air

You are extremely efficient, combining objectivity with practicality, and you are likely to be involved in your own health and health care, using conventional means of treatment for illness while being open to unorthodox methods. You plan and execute well and are in a positive to stay on top of a situation. Trouble results when you fall prey to skepticism, pessimism, or a cynical view of life.

Healing Mind, Body, Spirit

Earth/Water

You are simultaneously sensitive and grounded, both intuitive and practical. You have a talent for accepting whatever cards life deals to you and making them work. When ill, you tend to feel your way into your own depths to find the cure. Trouble results when you overindulge, which can produce addictions, or use your depths as a means of escape from harsh reality.

Air/Water

You are extremely sensitive, combining compassionate feelings with objectivity. You can detach from your emotions and empathetic responses and analyze your experience coolly. With both a logical mind and the ability to feel, you can effect the course of any illness from both angles. Trouble results when you rely too heavily on your intellectual abilities, which makes you high-strung and nervous.

Every person relates to each of the four elements differently, depending on their varying emphasis in the personality. For example, one person may be a "natural" swimmer, preferring to exercise in the water, sensing that the sea or lake shore acts as a restorative. Another is a "natural" runner, preferring to have the Earth firmly under his or her feet at all times and taking joy in the sights, sounds, and smells of the land beneath.

The elements refer to the most basic energies within us, essential dynamic life forces. The elemental makeup is the energy pattern of the individual. A grasp of these life principles and how they operate is a major step toward understanding what makes one ill and what will heal both physical and emotional disorders.

part three

The Transformative Healing Powers

chapter six
The Healing Body

ndemic in our own time is self-hate...a refusal of the ego to accept and work with what one happens to be.

~ Edward C. Whitmont, M.D.
The Alchemy of Healing

Healing Mind, Body, Spirit

As the vehicle of life, the body possesses its own inner wisdom and healing powers. Already they are at work within you all the time—repairing and replacing your cells, eliminating waste, nourishing tissues, fighting off germs, calming nerves, protecting from infection, balancing your hormones, and, when necessary, healing contusions and wounds. Most of the time you are almost completely unaware of all this activity. But you can control and accelerate your body's healing powers by learning to use them consciously.

Your body's healing power is as much a part of you, of your SELF, as your ability to think, to feel, to make decisions, to make love, to live. It's always there, on duty and on guard around-the-clock. You can think of it as an entire army, headed by a commanding general who supervises its operations. Each of your cells is a scientific genius, not only repairing itself, but having the capacity to renew and regenerate itself. In fact, every cell in your body replaces itself with a completely new cell every seven years. You literally produce a new body. Today, medical researchers are proving in the scientific laboratory what metaphysicians have known all along: *We can heal ourselves*. The SELF comes equipped with healing powers.

When things get seriously out of balance through stress or trauma, you can release the inner healing powers by conscious attention and effort. Note the word *attention*. It is the super key with which you can unlock your healing potential.

As you begin to move the power of your consciousness through yourself, you reach into the implicate order and activate the pattern of perfect health *already there* that puts you on the road to recovery. Of course, there will be times when standard-practice medical intervention will be necessary and useful. We aren't throwing the baby out with the bath water. But, conscious use of the techniques I will be describing can act both as preventive measures and as adjuncts to healing—whether or not an outside healer is involved.

The Healing Body

The life force is a powerful one. Just think of the fact that a tiny blade of grass, pushing up from a speck of a seed in the soil below, can crack open a cement sidewalk. The question arises: If we have such amazing restorative powers, why do we get sick?

There can be no completely definitive answer to that, but a large part of the reason is that we suffer from self-inflicted conditions, most often derived from negative and traumatic emotional experiences. These in turn afflict us with ongoing negative thought patterns, which often turn into illnesses.

Your body was made by a powerful force that has been making life forms, including the human body, for eons. This force lives within you, and it contains millions of years of wisdom. In the Hawaiian healing tradition called *Huna*, the body is said to have been created by your *unipihili*, which is your own personal elemental energy. This "entity" has created many bodies over time, for that is its work, and it does innumerable things for you—breathes, digests food, eliminates waste, warns you of imminent danger, runs your internal chemical production, puts you to sleep, wakes you up, and more.

Located in your solar plexus, your *unihipili* is the keeper of your personal archive, which is what the body is—the record of your life. Within its tissues are stored all of your experiences and memories. Becoming aware of your body and its needs and moods is the means to connect with your inner truth; that truth can set you free from illness. Your inner truth is revealed by your instincts.

Unfortunately, most of us have lost touch with the physical basis from which we derive. We ignore basic needs, override our natural drives with intellect or "willpower," allow ourselves to become emotionally stressed from a variety of causes—some minor, some major. Having lost respect for our basic instincts, which are always right, we fail to listen to our bodies. The way a person's body responds to stress of any kind is indicative of how and where the stress will manifest into illness or bodily disorder.

Unfortunately, in our science-oriented, technology-driven society we have lost our natural connection with the deep levels of wisdom within our bodies. We have lost the knowledge that our cells *are* basic intelligence organized into patterns both visible in the flesh and invisible in the inner reaches of our SELF.

By following the path of awareness, we can reconnect to this inner knowing. If you want to heal your body, first increase your level of awareness. Learn to heed the clues your body gives you and follow its directions no matter what the clock or anyone else tells you. Regaining communication with your body-self will put you on the road to health.

This is *not* a suggestion that we blame ourselves for getting sick. Most of the time we are not responsible for the negativity that comes our way, especially in childhood when many of the patterns that impact us negatively in later life are established. However, we *are* responsible for the maintenance of that negativity. Once we become aware of them, we can refuse to continue in the negative patterns that have caused ill health. Illness is a window of opportunity through which we can see clearly into our negative patterns and begin to transform them to conform to our true reality.

An example is my having a major surgical procedure, which I did not expect to survive. Not only did the illness that necessitated the operation push into my consciousness an awareness of the negative source, which promoted a healing of far-reaching dimensions, but it was the vehicle through which I finally learned the truth.

Because I believed my mother had died from reproductive-organ cancer, my doctor suspected a genetic link. He insisted that I obtain my mother's death certificate so that he could know the exact organic site of her cancer. Guess what? She died of carcinoma of the *stomach*. And so, after carrying a burden of guilt for thirty years, I learned that my birth had nothing at all to do with her death!

I reveal this personal information in case you are resistant to the idea that past emotional trauma directly correlates to physical illness. My endometriosis was a clear one-to-one instance of this.

Since we are talking here about self-healing, the question arises: could I have healed myself without surgical intervention? Probably not at the physical level, considering the advanced stage of the disease when it was discovered. Had I known earlier what I know now, I might have avoided the disease, but my sense of it is that the disease was *purposeful*. Had it not occurred, I might never have known how my mother actually died nor been able to absolve myself of the unconscious guilt that had so deeply poisoned my life. My illness was an important factor in my ultimate journey toward wholeness. Afterward, when my physical body had returned to health, I began to live more in accordance with who I am. Also, whereas many women with endometriosis suffer from it all their lives, after five symptom-free years my doctor pronounced me completely cured of the disease. However, my real healing took place at a much deeper level than mere flesh describes, enabling me to develop a broader perspective with which to handle my life. I hope to enable you to develop a perspective which will render you better able to cope with present illness and past trauma. I do not claim that this is an easy or automatic process. There are those who become ill and are "cured" by the medical establishment but who do not sustain healing at the deep, implicate-order level. Those who suffer chronic illness fall into this category, as has been shown by recent research.

The body also tends to symbolize illness through the affected parts. For example, during my writer's-block crisis, mystified by the out-of-the-blue occurrence of intense but apparently causeless pain in my left arm, I analyzed it symbolically: left arm = right brain, or feeling and intuitive nature; unable to use arm = *disarmed*. Conclusion: my *feeling* state was rendering me powerless. My emotional response was weighting the scale all to one side, preventing my logical, left brain from doing its job. Detachment was needed to restore the balance. This understanding served first to ameliorate the pain and, finally, when I had put the insight into action through releasing meditations, to remove it completely.

Some conditions are less easy to analyze, but chronic stiffness, for example, indicates something within that is restricted and needs to be released. Breast cancer is thought to be related to the nurturing a woman both gives and has received, or—most often—has not received. And so on. Even accidents can be seen to have causal roots in the unconscious matrix if one looks closely enough. A broken arm can serve a psychological purpose.

Following, we will be examining and exploring various healing "powers" that you already have inherent in your SELF. Each plan contains information about how you can activate healing on the implicate-order plane through the use of relaxation exercises, visualizations, and meditations. As you practice these exercises, you will be releasing the healer within by activating the healthy, positive qualities of your SELF—body, mind, and spirit. No matter what you want to heal at this moment, as you begin the healing process and devote yourself to it, you will experience the "magic" of connectedness.

The Healing Power of Breath

Breath is life. When breath stops, life stops. The vital force of life comes into our bodies with our breath. Yet, we are mostly unaware of this and often neglect to breathe fully and deeply. Breath is the gateway to improved health and to amplified healing. It is something we take for granted, for we could hardly function if we had to consciously remember to breathe. Yet most of us are rarely aware of our breathing until it becomes impaired, by a cold or by shortness of breath. When we become aware of our breathing, we connect to the implicate order or realm of subtle energies within us. Breath is the link we have to our unconscious selves; it is the carrier not only of oxygen but of information about our inner states. Awareness and control of breath allow us to consciously open ourselves to our innate healing powers.

Although Western medicine has largely ignored the benefits of conscious breathing, most Eastern philosophies teach that we live in a sea of vital energy—and that we absorb and activate this with our breath. The Hindu yogi tradition calls this energy *prana*. Oriental mind-body balancing techniques, such as acupuncture and shiatzu, refer to this vital force as *Qi* (chi). The Hawaiian Huna tradition calls it *mana* (*mana loa* in its highest form). In Hawaiian, the word for "to think" is *mana-o*.

Not only is this subtle energy in the very air we breathe, it also circulates through our bodies along specific channels called *meridians*. These are mapped along twelve courses, or channels, in the body. Imbalances in the energy flowing along these lines are believed to be the cause of illness.

Controlled breathing permits us to extract new energy from the air. Our physical bodies can store this energy in the same way food is stored as fat. When this subtle energy is in short supply, you feel down, listless, tired, and you can get sick. When it is in abundant supply, you feel "up," energized, optimistic, and full of energy. Though the energy is subtle, it is very real.

You can prove this to yourself by paying attention to the ion content of the air you breathe. Air is charged with positive and negative ions, and a surplus of the former results in an oppressively heavy atmosphere, like that before a thunderstorm. Positive ions sap our energy. Think of how you feel when a storm is brewing and the sky lowers darkly. Negative ions release uplifting energy into the air. When the storm breaks and the rain comes pelting down, the air is cleared and refreshed. Your spirits lift and your mood brightens. You feel energized and ready to go. Proper deep breathing has the effect of saturating your system with negative ions, contributing to release of tension and to mental calmness.

The energy of breath can be used to repel invading germs, to mend broken bones, to close wounds, to calm the mind, to soothe upset emotions. Here are some affirmations you can use to activate the healing power in your breath.

My breathing connects me to all parts of myself.
Breath is my source, linking body, mind, and spirit.
I now consciously breathe in the vital life force.

Breathing Healing Energy

This is a simple exercise designed to enable you to increase the vital force in your body in order to combat illness or effect healing. It can also be used anytime you are tired and need to refresh yourself. You can do this almost anywhere—sitting quietly at home, in your car, on a train. In the middle of a bustling city, I slip into a church, sit in a back pew, and breathe in energy.

Relax and close your eyes. Tell yourself that you are now going to add vital energy every time you inhale deeply. Think of it as putting extra dollars into your energy bank for use whenever you need it. Realize that you are always surrounded by this vital healing force, that it sustains and nourishes you all the time, even when you are unaware of it.

Begin to breathe slowly and rhythmically, not altering your breath pattern but simply becoming

> aware of it. Now, begin to breathe deeply—slowly and deeply. As you inhale each breath, be aware of the energy coming into your body. Imagine it filling up all the cells of your body like you would fill a balloon by blowing air into it. Let the sense of being filled with energy spread throughout your body. Feel it energize your mind. Hold each breath for a few seconds while you imagine these results. Then, as you exhale, feel the energy being retained within you. Let the breath go out smoothly and easily. Do not force or strain.

Most adults are shallow breathers. They sip the air the way a Victorian lady sipped her cup of tea, and for the same reason—not to appear coarse. Taking in generous amounts of air seems impolite to many people, especially those who feel socially restricted and insecure about how others will view them. A good belly breath, like a good belly laugh, seems not to belong in polite company.

Breath, like food, nourishes our every cell, and cleanses our blood. But we insist on starving ourselves of this vital nutrient. The good news is that changing breathing patterns is easy. Anyone can do it. Changing your breathing starts with becoming aware of it. Learning this skill is extremely easy.

Abdominal, or diaphragmatic, breathing is belly breathing. When the air is taken in, the diaphragm contracts and the abdomen expands; when the air is exhaled, the reverse occurs. To practice abdominal breathing, imagine that your in-breath is filling a balloon in your belly. When the balloon is full, exhale until you feel it is completely empty. Just a few of these deep abdominal breaths will bring relief from tension—and half of pain is tension.

Breathing for Pain

Do this exercise when you are in pain. First, take as comfortable a position as you can manage, preferably lying down. Then, consciously shift your breathing into abdominal breathing by taking a deep breath and letting it go with a sigh of relief. Next, feel the next several breaths enter your belly and fill the "balloon" there. Exhale fully each time. Finally, begin to *breathe into the pain*. Feel the breath going deep into the area of your body that feels pain. Continue this until you feel a sense of relaxation. This is often felt as an internal "shift," like shifting the gears of a car.

Being aware of your breathing patterns develops a communications link between the conscious and the unconscious, between body and mind, between spirit and psyche. Adding the factor of imagination increases the benefit. The following is a yoga exercise known as "polarization."

Breathing with Color

To do this exercise, lie face up in a comfortable position, either on your bed or on a mat on the floor. Align your body, with feet pointing south and head north, to the Earth's magnetic field. Let your palms rest face up with the arms stretched out alongside the body. Begin breathing as described above, slowly and rhythmically, and as you breathe, breathe in one *color* and exhale another. If you breathe in a warm color, breathe out a cool color, and vice versa. If you want to energize yourself, breathe in a warm color such as red, the strongest; orange, which enlivens; or yellow, which promotes optimism. Breathe out a cool color, such as blue or green. For a calming or relaxing effect, do the opposite. Breathe in a cool color and breathe out a warm color. Think of the incoming breath as a positive current, the outgoing breath as a negative current. By breathing in these two polar opposites, you are balancing your energy state toward health. Imagine these polarized currents circulating through your body, one after the other, cleansing and purifying, healing and revivifying.

Deep breathing is not only a powerful transformative healing power on its own, it is also fundamental to all the healing powers discussed in this book.

The Healing Power of Relaxation

We all know that tension and stress cause illness, from the minor aching of stiff muscles to heart and circulatory problems. Yet, relaxation seems to evade us most of the time. Why? The answer is not completely clear, but clues can be found in our outlook on life. When we look upon life as an adversary or threat, we are in a perpetual state of "fight or flight." Instead of releasing the tension when danger is past, we store it; the retention results in a dangerous build-up that can bring on stress-related disease, such as high blood pressure, ulcers, and the like.

In the late 1960s, Harvard cardiologist Herbert Benson, M.D., was involved in some physiologic tests on meditators. He discovered that relaxation methods, of which there are many, caused both psychological and *physiological* changes that served to counterbalance the body's response to "fight or flight." He called this the "relaxation response." Not a technique but a coordinated series of internal changes occurring when the mind and body become calm and tranquil, the relaxation response can be achieved by numerous means, such as deep breathing, muscle relaxation, meditation, visualizations, and prayer. The simplest of these is called "focused meditation."

As described by Benson, the relaxation response exercise consists of two parts: one, repetition of a word, sound, prayer, or phrase; two, passive disregard of everyday thoughts that come to mind. This is continued for ten to twenty minutes and practiced once or twice each day.

Benson showed that the relaxation response caused bodily transformations. Heart rate, breathing rate, muscle tension, and oxygen consumption fall below resting levels; blood pressure can decrease; and the waking brain shifts into the slower patterns associated with reverie and daydreaming. These slightly altered states of consciousness promote healing in the same way sleep does.

In other studies, insomnia patients who elicited the relaxation response regularly were able to sleep better and return to normal sleep patterns; chronic pain patients were able to decrease their doctor visits by one-third; patients with hypertension were able to lower their blood pressure; and psychologist Ann Webster, Ph.D., who teaches the relaxation response to patients with cancer and AIDS, has shown that these techniques reduce anticipatory nausea in those being treated with chemotherapy. Another Harvard study showed a reduction of severe PMS symptoms by 58 percent.

Physical relaxation is an important adjunct to the healing process; consistent practice is a wonderful preventive measure. There are two basic types of physical relaxation—*sequential* and *tension*. In sequential relaxation, you focus on each part of your body separately, from the toes up, allowing it to become limp and flaccid before moving on to the next part. In tension relaxation, you tense and release each muscle or muscle group in turn. Below are exercises for both types. Here are some relaxing affirmations you can use.

I now relax and let go of all tension, worry, and disease.
I now allow myself to relax totally into peace.
My body and mind are now fully relaxed into spirit.

Sequential Technique

To do this, lie comfortably on the floor or on a bed and breathe deeply several times, consciously inhaling fresh energy and consciously exhaling all negative tension. Then, starting with your toes, focus on each part of your body in turn: feet, ankles, calves, knees, thighs, hips, lower back, upper back, abdomen, chest, arms, hands, neck, spine, head. As you do this, mentally instruct each part to relax completely, and linger until you feel your muscles loosen. Tell each set of muscles to go limp, and feel yourself gradually sinking into an inert state of being. When you have finished with this sequence, do it in reverse, from head to toes.

Tense-and-Relax Technique

This is known as "progressive" relaxation. It was developed by Dr. Edmund Jacobson, an American physician, whose research into muscle physiology and relaxation gained him worldwide fame and set the groundwork for other psychotherapeutic techniques based on relaxation, such as natural childbirth. Yogis and traditional practitioners have used similar methods for hundreds of years. Here is the basic method.

To do this exercise, choose a time and place where you can be alone and quiet for at least thirty minutes. Prepare your environment by lighting a candle, playing soft music, scenting the air, or anything else that appeals to you as an atmosphere in which to relax completely.

Sit comfortably in a chair or lie down on the floor or a bed. You are going to progressively tense-and-relax each of the major muscle groups of your whole body, beginning with the feet. Take a deep breath, let it out slowly, and gradually tense the muscles in your feet. Do this cautiously, because feet and legs tends to cramp. Hold the tension for a count of three. Relax, tighten again, relax. Repeat this a third time. Leaving the foot relaxed, move up to the calf muscles and repeat the three-time procedure. Continue up to the thighs, the abdominal muscles, the buttocks, each time in sets of three. Proceed to your chest, arms, hands—tighten, relax, tighten, relax, tighten, relax. Next, go to your neck and shoulders. Move up to your face and make a "monster face" with open mouth and stretched muscles. This is known in yoga as the "lion face," and it is used to prevent wrinkles and sagging face muscles. Last, squeeze your eyes tightly and then relax them completely three times. You should now be completely relaxed. Remain still for a few minutes, enjoying this state of being.

Breathing Relaxation

This is a simple technique that takes only a little time. Sit or lie down in a safe and comfortable spot with no distractions. Loosen any tight clothing, unbutton or untie anything that is restrictive on your body. Begin to breath *consciously*, following your breath in and out of your lungs. Breathe in through the nostrils, out through the mouth. Pay full attention to your breath, in and out, in and out. Listen to the sound, and feel the rhythmic pulsing of it. Continue this until you begin to feel calm and relaxed, a state usually signaled by the breath becoming slow and even.

You can deepen your relaxation using breath by imagining that you are breathing in *prana*, or the vital force of life, and exhaling all tension and negative feeling or experience. One way to do this is to choose a color for both the *prana* and the negative energy. See a stream of one color (positive) coming into your body as you inhale, and see a stream of the other color (negative) flowing out of you as you exhale. White and black are easy—white is the pure energy of light, while black represents any dark thoughts. But feel free to use any color that represents to you healing energy and release of negative energy. Don't worry if distracting thoughts arise; you can tell them you will attend to their needs later. Let them float off like soap bubbles in the air, and return to attending your breathing.

Instant Mini-Relaxation

Once you have fully experienced relaxation using one of these techniques and fixed this sensation firmly in your mind as a mental picture, you can achieve instant relaxation simply by calling up the image you have created of your totally relaxed self. To do this, take a comfortable position and remember what it felt like to be completely relaxed. Your subconscious

> mind remembers everything. Tell it that you are now going to take ten deep breaths, and that when you have finished you will be as completely relaxed as when you went through the entire relaxation process previously. Then, slowly and gently begin to breathe, counting to ten breaths. If you like, for deeper relaxation, you can extend this to twenty breaths, but be sure to stipulate to your subconscious what you intend to do. When you have finished the number of breaths you fixed in advance, you will feel relaxed and refreshed. Use this method frequently throughout the day.

As we have seen, relaxation transforms us physiologically as well as psychologically. It is also the gateway to the use of the other healing powers to be discussed.

The Healing Power of Touch

Although there are many healing techniques that are based on touch, such as massage, chiropractic, and the laying on of hands, you do not need another person to use the healing power of touch. Unfortunately, most of us have been taught that touching ourselves is narcissistic or, worse, sinful. The result is that we touch ourselves only perfunctorily—as in the performance of personal hygiene—or furtively, in an erotic manner. We need to learn the healing power of touch because it is one of the easiest and most effective of healing tools.

Touching yourself in a loving and healing way can be an extremely positive experience, and since tactile experience is so fundamental, self-touch is an excellent avenue into the implicate order. Touching yourself can be a meditative experience, whether it is sexually neutral or erotic, and it can be combined with the use of words. Joan Borysenko, in *The Power of the Mind to Heal*, tells of how her child cured a painful plantar wart by holding the affected foot in his hands and saying, "Begone, wart, begone."

You can also practice your healing touch on other people and animals—even plants can benefit from your loving touch. This spring, an amaryllis in my study that annually produces glorious apricot-colored blossoms put out its two-foot-long prebloom fronds, which collapsed at a right angle to the bulb. Taking them in my hands, I stroked them upward for several minutes, and the next day they were standing erect on their own. Such is the power of touch combined with genuine caring.

Having had experience with hands-on healing of others, I devised self-touch as a means to alleviate the excruciating muscle cramps of my own post-polio syndrome. After struggling with this problem for a long time, I began to practice the healing power of touch on myself. When a cramp struck, I'd gently stroke or rub the limb that was in agony and say, "You are now relaxed." The pain that could often mean a night of misery can now be alleviated in a short time, and as I have continued to use the power of touch, the cramps have become much less frequent.

Every mother uses the healing power of touch whenever she kisses a small hurt "to make it better." And every loved child knows that mummy's kiss has tremendous healing power. You can kiss yourself to make it well. Here are some affirmations you can use.

My hands have healing power and I use them in love.
My love-filled touch now alleviates my pain.
With this touch, I thee love and heal.

Letting Go of Self-Consciousness

To use the healing power of touch—that is, to touch yourself positively—you must first let go of any feeling of embarrassment about putting your hands on your own body. To begin, wash your hands and face thoroughly with a sweet-smelling soap, and dry them on a soft, warm towel. You want to maximize the tactile experience in every way possible, and that means using your other senses as well. Next, put some lotion on your hands and rub them together until they are warm. Then, gently begin to stroke and caress your face, saying either silently or aloud, "I love you, you're beautiful" or other words of affection and praise. (Men should shave first.) Spend ten minutes stroking your face, and then look in the mirror at the lovely glow.

One of my favorite forms of meditative self-touch can be done in the shower by consciously stroking any body part that is tense, in pain, or about which you feel negative. Speak words of love and healing to it. Learning to cherish all parts of your body is a powerful healing tool. You can do this outside the shower as well—standing, sitting, or lying down. Before sleep is a good time to practice self-touch, especially if something hurts. Even if you can't reach the hurting part, such as your back, you can stroke the areas of your body that you can reach and allow the *intention* to heal to penetrate into the implicate order. You will find this a very soothing experience, and the more you use it the more effective it will become.

Learning to Cherish Yourself

You can use this healing power to help heal any illness or pain. Stroking yourself gently while saying or thinking loving words can work wonders.

Use this technique especially to reunite yourself to parts of your body that you have denied or despised. Because we are fed manufactured idealized images of beauty or masculinity, we learn to think of our bodies as inadequate or inferior. Women especially are afflicted by this. Surveys show that even pre-teenaged girls already "hate" their hips, thighs, breasts. Until women develop the good sense to reject these idealized images—and to teach their daughters to reject them as well—the noxious fumes they exude will continue to permeate our psyches.

However, you can take steps to heal the old pains you have suffered because your body didn't fit the image-makers' ideal. Touch any part of you that you consider imperfect or a problem and *give love to it*. It's the only body you have, and it deserves your kind and loving care and concern.

The transformative power of touch can be dramatic indeed. For example, babies fail to develop properly unless they are touched, held, and handled. Various body therapies can release deep-seated, tightly held, emotional pain by the use of touch alone, and the mere touch of a hand when one is in distress can bring instant relief and comfort. Give yourself the gift of loving touch—and give it to others.

~ *Healing Mind, Body, Spirit*

~ The Healing Power of Rest

One might think the healing power of *rest* would be considered a given. "Bedrest" is perhaps the most frequent prescription for everything from a cold to a wrenched back. Yet, oddly, true rest eludes most of us. We sleep—and wake tired. We vacation—and return home exhausted. Why is this?

Rest is an *attitude*. It is giving yourself permission to be quiet, free of demands—your own or others. It is a place *within*. Although meditation can lead to rest or be an adjunct to it, it is not actually rest. When you are truly resting, you have no place to go, nothing to do, nothing to accomplish. You are utterly at peace within yourself—at rest. It is a state of calm emptiness, like the still point at the hub of the turning wheel. Life goes on all around us all the time, but we can withdraw into that center where all is still and unmoving and there gain our deserved rest.

Rest, though it refreshes us for what we must do, is not an interim to prepare you for another day's work. It is a *state of being*. When you rest, you activate your inner healing powers. It is a place where you reconnect with your SELF, with your deep internal rhythms, with your inner wisdom that knows how to heal you and balance you.

No, rest isn't a given. It's a commodity in increasingly short supply in our busy lives. Those "busy lives" are usually something we are quite proud of—as if overfilled hours, days, weeks, months, years, and lives earned extra credit in heaven.

Recently, while attending a funeral, I heard one mourner say, "That's why I keep myself so busy—you never know when you'll die." Whereas the latter statement is true, the former may hasten its arrival. Those who cannot rest, or who refuse rest, set themselves up for all sorts of ailments. Rest is natural—as natural as breathing—but, just as many people don't breathe deeply and fully, many of us have lost the ability to rest, forfeited the knowledge of how rest is made. The very word *restful* has a soothing, calming sound to it. Think of a restful day and see what comes to mind.

Many people think the need for rest is a weakness, a lower-level activity that must be endured in order to get back to work or other pursuits. Rest is the glue that holds body, mind, and spirit together. You know that when you are tired you tend to "come apart." Tired children are fretful, prone to accidents and tears. Tired adults are grumpy, short-tempered, prone to argument and emotional upsets. When I'm tired I find I can't do simple things well. Though I am an experienced and accomplished cook, I know that when I am tired I'll cut or burn myself.

Tired people make mistakes, injure themselves and others, and become ill. You've heard the saying "I'm just bone tired." That is what happens when we fail to get proper rest. We are tired right down to the marrow of our bones. Lack of genuine rest is a major factor in stress-related illnesses, for our bodies (and minds and spirits) do not get the chance to recuperate fully from the daily wear and tear. Like a stretched-out rubber band, they lose the ability to "bounce back."

Others confuse rest with laziness. "Doing nothing" is considered to be some kind of minor crime associated with a bad character. Can you comfortably reply "Nothing" to the question "What are you doing?" Or do you have to invent some activity in which you were supposedly engaged? In our Puritan-based culture, doing nothing is a dangerous condition, a situation not to be tolerated. We've all had "Idle hands are the devil's workshop," drummed into us when we were children.

As adults, we don't have anyone over us to perpetuate the notion that rest is somehow connected with evil—that it engenders "impure thoughts" or mischievous actions—but we enforce the dictum on ourselves all the same. The busy housewife feels guilty if she collapses on the sofa for half an hour with her feet up. If interrupted, she is quick to assume a pose of industriousness. Office workers use their lunch time to

༄ Healing Mind, Body, Spirit

go shopping or perform errands. The idea of doing "nothing" seems to equate to *being* nothing, as if, instead of "I think, therefore I am," the motto were "I do, therefore I am." That "nothing" is a valuable place, one you need to develop and protect. It is a refuge in times of stress; a sacred space within yourself; a source of strength, joy, and healing.

Only you can know what rests *you*. Rest means different things to different people. Your healing type can be a guide to what will give you authentic rest. It might be fishing on a lake, hiking up a mountain, petting your cat, or cooking a meal. Rest does not necessarily mean lack of activity, but must include some cessation of it. Perhaps after the hike up the mountain you sit quietly for hours and contemplate the vast emptiness of the cloudless blue sky. For me, rest takes many forms; the experience of altered states of consciousness is one of my favorites. Remember, rest is a profound place within yourself. You must find it and identify it and experience it on your own.

There is currently a vogue in the mind-body health community for "mindfulness," a Buddhist concept that has been Americanized. While the conscious practice of being mindful on a moment-to-moment basis benefits some, others report it causes anxiety, worry, and strain—"Am I doing it right?" You'll never have to ask yourself if you are "doing it right" when you have found your place of rest. You'll *know*. Here are some restful affirmations you can use.

> *I now rest in the spirit where all is free and calm.*
> *I now rest in solitude, comfort, and safety within.*
> *Rest is my right, and I embrace it with all my being.*

"Mindless" Meditation

Here is a meditation I've devised to put you into a state of mind that can lead to real rest. To do this meditation—which is really not a meditation at all in any formal sense—recline or lie down comfortably when you can be alone and uninterrupted for an hour. Turn lights down or off and eliminate outside noises and distractions. Close your eyes and let yourself experience the silence around you, and then move inward and find a place of silence inside. Let yourself stay in this place as long as you feel comfortable. Begin to follow your breath without trying to alter it. Just feel the quiet rhythm of your SELF. As you do this, let your mind wander wherever it wants to go, like a puppy let outside for an airing. Follow it if you wish to see what interests it, but make no judgments. Think of your mind as a butterfly lighting now on one flower, now on another, gathering nectar. Don't push or move your mind in any particular direction. *Let it go where it wants*. That is the key here. So much meditation tries to harness the mind, to tether it like a goat on a rope as bait for large game. Don't do that. As your mind is given the freedom to roam here and there, to *play* at will, it will lead you to your place of rest.

Deep and genuine rest is transformative in many ways. It opens us up to our larger possibilities, which can remain remote or hidden during ordinary waking states characterized by busyness and activity. Being in a state of true rest connects us to our intuitive levels and the implicate pattern of health and well-being residing in our SELF.

The Healing Power of Openness

So many illnesses result from constriction and repression. Stomach cramps are produced by fear and anxiety, rheumatic stiffness symbolizes an unbending attitude. One can often see this facially or in body language.

What happens is that the inner pattern of stiffness and constraint works itself out bodily, becoming innervation; constricted movements and behaviors; and illness, especially chronic pain. Closing one's self off to the gamut of humanity's multiplicity means living in a state of perennial constriction and isolation, with concomitant results. For example, a pattern of dogmatic self-righteousness and emotional denial can concur with cardiac and circulatory malfunction, such as the aptly named "hardening of the arteries," which often precedes cardiac arrest.

Opening ourselves to the vast possibilities inherent in our own natures releases great healing power. Intellectual openness to alternative treatment is important if we are to access all available means to treat ourselves when we fall ill, but more important is emotional openness to our own SELF and its healing abilities.

I devised the "lotus" meditation that follows for those suffering from what I call "concretized" thoughts, emotions, and attitudes. So often we harm ourselves by our refusal to open up to new possibilities. A widow I know almost starved herself by maintaining that she "didn't know how" to cook for one person. Having spent a lifetime preparing meals for her husband and children, when she found herself alone she would not cook nutritious food for herself. No matter how many suggestions I made about meals-for-one or how many tantalizing recipes I provided, she refused to open to the possibility that she could change a lifelong attitude that insisted all cooking be done in large quantities. Eventually, she became quite ill and was hospitalized for internal complications brought on by malnutrition, which could have been avoided. Here are some affirmations you can use.

I open fully to the healing power within myself.
Spirit flows through me in a healing stream.
All obstacles to healing are now and forever removed.

Lotus Meditation

Prepare for this meditation by choosing a quiet place you can be alone and comfortable for half an hour. If possible, first relax in a warm bath scented and softened with salts or oil. This meditation is best done without clothes or only lightly clad or covered, preferably in white. Light a white candle and arrange yourself in a comfortable position lying down or reclining. If the air is cool, cover yourself; if warm, remain nude.

Now, breathe slowly and deeply several times and allow your body to relax completely. Imagine yourself a seed at the bottom of a deep pool where all is dark and tranquil. Feel yourself begin to put out roots into the nourishing bottom and anchor yourself there. Next, feel a stem begin to grow up and out of you, reaching upward for the light above. Feel it move through the abyssal water until it breaks the surface. Then, feel yourself putting out little new leaves on the surface of the water, stretching in all directions.

As these leaves grow larger and stronger, feel yourself growing into the bud of a beautiful lotus. Let this bud rest on the surface, in the light, for a few minutes, and then—slowly—begin to open up your petals, one by one, until you have unfurled a glorious blossom, fully opened and gently floating on its undulant stem, but firmly rooted in the earth at the bottom of the pond. Feel the light on your petals, soak up the warmth of the sun, breathe in the cool of the

Healing Mind, Body, Spirit

air. Say, "I am open. I am open. I now open fully to all my possibilities. I open to my inner healing powers. I release and let go all constraints, restrictions, limits. Whatever comes, I welcome. My openness brings happiness, pleasure, reward, and healing. I remain open to the light at all times. My roots are strong so I have no fear of being open. My state of openness brings me all good things."

Remain with this feeling of being totally, safely, and completely open for as long as the feeling lasts. When it begins to fade, *slowly* return to waking consciousness by breathing gently and easily, continuing to feel yourself as open to your inner possibilities, for healing and for bringing all good things into your life. When you open your eyes, remember the feeling of calm confidence you experienced in the open state.

Rest quietly until you feel yourself retracting into the bud state. Now that your lotus self has blossomed fully, you know you can always open when you wish. You do not need to be fully open all of the time—you can rest in the bud state, or even return to the seed state to gather new force.

The goal is to be *able* to open fully to the transformative process of self-healing. Carry this awareness with you as you progress through the healing powers that come next.

chapter seven
The Healing Mind

Just as scientists have found that positive beliefs can engender wellness, they also have found that negative beliefs and influences can induce illness.... The brain sends messages throughout the body via neurotransmitters that signal the body to respond as if the thought were a real event.

~ Herbert Benson, M.D.
Timeless Healing

We all know people who literally "make themselves sick," with uncontrolled outbursts of emotion—usually anger, hate, fear, or envy. The stereotypical figure of the person engorged with fury suddenly dying of apoplexy is not so far from truth. *Overexpression* of emotions means identifying with them, a dangerous state that clouds the mind's ability to make rational decisions.

Unexpressed, or repressed, emotions are also a major cause of illness. Bottled-up resentment, frustrations, and seething rage all put the entire system under tension and stress, with the effect of weakening the immune system and impeding function of the organs. Keeping emotions repressed diverts a tremendous amount of life energy from its proper function of maintaining our health and happiness.

At the other end of the spectrum lies *denial*, the refusal to acknowledge painful feelings. Those in denial stoutly maintain that everything is A-OK, no matter what the evidence suggests. This shutting off of the flow of feelings is linked to a number of illnesses, from migraine headaches to chronic back pain. These often can be analyzed symbolically. People with headaches don't want to *think* about the problem; irritable bowel syndrome cries out, "I can't *eliminate* these feelings."

Although the conscious mind remains unaware of the unexpressed emotion, the unconscious is all too painfully aware, and it reacts accordingly. Since the person refuses to acknowledge the painful emotion, it is somatized into a bodily state where it cannot be ignored. Through this process, illness can be seen as the product of wrong thoughts, beliefs, and emotions. These negative forces infiltrate the body, restricting and damaging the life force.

This is not, however, to say that chronic disease is simply a matter of repressed emotion; nor that it is a result of conscious choice. The idea here is that the emotional content serves to obstruct healing. While some patients may deliberately malinger in order to get attention, staying sick for what psychologists call "secondary gains," these secondary gains are usually not consciously sought but are a product of the totality of the person's psychology. This is not to suggest a one-to-one, cause-and-effect relationship, for the complexity of the human organism does not allow that interpretation. Simplistic formulations do not get at the enormous subtlety and intricacy of the mind-body-spirit relationship, and each instance must be investigated individually.

Nonetheless, in many cases it is possible to see connections, whether direct or indirect, actual or symbolic, between illness and its ultimate source. To do so is to realize that physical intervention—no matter how initially successful—will not lead to real healing unless changes in the mental realm are also accomplished. It is the very fact that healing can be blocked by the mind that offers the possibility of treatment.

While we may not be able to heal ourselves beyond what is physically possible, nor speed up the natural rate at which healing can occur, we can help the process along by recognizing the role our thoughts and emotions play in any illness. In this manner, we can proceed to consciously improve our healing by removing obstacles to it, providing it with missing information, and incorporating into it our sense of wholeness, for it is the whole person who is ill and only restoration of wholeness can bring healing.

A single thread runs through all preindustrial approaches to healing. It is the concept of illness as a *dis-ease*—an imbalance in the person's relationship to the SELF and, by extension, to the cosmos. One must address the *totality* of the person and the environment in order to effect the healing. The *allopathic*, or standard Western practice of medicine, does not usually consider the emotional or temperamental factor in illness, unless the diagnosis is "It's all in your head." This is because the scientifically trained mind-set seems to fear that admitting into conscious practice anything not clearly identifiable in the laboratory, and replicable by experiment, will immediately regress them to the darkest of the Dark Ages, where superstition and mumbo jumbo passed for medicine.

Seventy years ago Dr. Alexis Carrel, in *Man the Unknown*, wrote that "Envy, hate, and fear, when these sentiments are habitual, are capable of starting organic changes and genuine disease." Catharine Ponder, author of several books on healing, says, "When you change those negative beliefs and emotions, you change the body which houses them in its cells." She further postulates that there are "thought centers," which settle in various parts of the body, affecting it according to whether they are charged negatively or positively.

Recent major studies show that as many as 75 percent of visits to doctors are for "self-limiting" illnesses that will improve without intervention, or for anxiety and stress-related problems. According to Joan Borysenko in *Minding the Body, Mending the Mind*, restoring the entire system's natural balance is the way to promote healing, but many therapies "have failed because they address only the physical symptoms rather than the underlying causes." Borysenko goes on to assert that,

> The underlying issues have as much to do with the meaning of life as with learning to use the power of the mind to reduce symptoms....[W]e are already perfect—our essential core is peaceful and whole. The work of healing is in peeling away the barriers of fear and past conditioning that keep us unaware of our true nature of wholeness and love....Discovering the peaceful inner core, in turn, brings the body back to wholeness or allows us to live well in spite of our physical limitations.

Though the superbly healthy may not consider inner peace to be a factor in healing, it is essential to the process of transformation I have been describing. With peace of mind, we can advance fearlessly into our new and larger selves and be enriched by our experiences on the healing journey. As we travel the path of self-transformation, we free ourselves from the impact of negative states of mind such as fear and resentment, anger and apathy, grief and loneliness. As we pass through the necessary stages with compassion and determination, we reach the goal of inner peacefulness and are healed. In *Healing Mind, Healthy Woman*, Alice D. Domar, Ph.D., says,

> Each mind-body method is a way to cultivate peace of mind. Each is a pathway to a spacious inner ground where seeds of well-being can be planted, germinate, and grow. Once we inhabit this ground, we can still be hurt but we can't be spiritually destroyed by illness or infirmity.

Thomas Edison said, "Every cell thinks," and current scientific effort is beginning to confirm this. Quantum physics is showing that we live in an "intelligent universe," which constantly transmits and receives information from and to all its parts. As a consequence, "life" creates its dynamic processes based on the information it receives and to which it responds. The same is true of your body-mind-spirit. By changing the messages and the quality of the information being input, you can change the output, improving your health and your life.

It is clear, however, that we must be willing to make changes, to adapt ourselves to the transforming process. Those who, rather than altering their mind-set, remain in the same "space," refusing to find new attitudes, may be "cured," but the cure will be superficial. Heart bypass surgery cannot correct the hardening of the spiritual arteries nor force a rigid, power-motivated "Type A" person to change his or her ways of encountering life. Those who resist the transforming power of the SELF and march to the drumbeat of Ego alone—a tune called most often by exalted expectations and societal standards—can never truly be cured, nor saved.

Attitude is all. The person who is ego-bent upon maintaining an old and outworn stance in the face of urgent need for change and for shucking off negative patterns—or even positive ones that have outlived their usefulness—will ultimately face an impasse where no choice is left. The driven, materialistic personality, hell-bent on collecting as much gain and goods as the world allows, may, after a heart attack has been successfully dealt with, suffer a lethal stroke. Refusal to "give in" to the needed change, on an inner as well as outer level, or an unwillingness to accept changing circumstances around you, can lead to a biological imbalance, weakening the immune system and permitting disease to manifest. As the sixteenth-century philosopher-physician Paracelsus wrote, "The curative power of medicines often consist not so much in the spirit that is hidden in them, as in the spirit in which they are taken."

The Healing Power of Grief

The *failure to grieve* causes many problems. Often, when one of a long-married pair dies, the other, though not ill, follows in short order. Yet, grief is actually one of the most powerful fuels of transformation, but only by allowing ourselves to go through the entire process do we reap the benefits. When we fail to mourn, it's as if a part of us gets frozen in time. Frozen grief freezes other emotions as well—it robs us of the capacity to feel joy, to relish simple pleasures, to love freely. Unresolved, it can turn into chronic low-grade depression that saps emotional, mental, and physical energy.

Unfortunately, our culture provides little support for the grief process. Rituals of mourning have become truncated, or abandoned altogether as being old-fashioned, out-of-date, slightly embarrassing reminders of the "old country." Or, if we are of the Puritan tradition, we consider prolonged grief to be something of a moral failing. The mourner is advised to get on with life. But grief must be experienced fully in order to move on to the next stage of growth.

Studies of the psychology of cancer patients discovered that many had suffered a major loss or setback from six months to two years prior to the onset of the disease. These people had not grieved their losses but had translated them into illness.

One particularly difficult situation is when the person has not gone through the normal grieving process. A client of mine was widowed suddenly when she was barely thirty, but the needs and demands of her four children forced her to shelve her grief, which lay untended for many years until she developed a lung condition. In therapy with me, she realized her lungs were clogged from "stuffed" emotions and feelings that had never been "aired"—making it almost impossible for her to breathe. I guided her through the grieving process described here and she improved in a remarkably short time.

Fortunately, we can put ourselves through the grieving process consciously, even if it is long after the fact, as I did in the wake of endometriosis and chronic fatigue syndrome. In the first instance I was deprived of going through the process of grief for my mother, partly because she died when I was a baby, partly because my father, stuck in his anger about her death, deliberately obliterated all evidence of her life, I had unknowingly carried that noxious burden deep within until I got sick and subsequently realized the need to mourn my deep loss. In the second instance, I had failed to accept a grievous emotional loss as a fact of life, clinging unrealistically to the unconscious hope that what I lost would somehow be returned to me. This understanding was key to my ultimate healing.

In the absence of social support, we are usually left alone with our grief. Others, uncomfortable around both illness and death, don't know what to say, and though they may want to help, they also want to believe that disease (and even death) can be avoided, or easily remedied.

Grief, no matter how painful it seems at first, is nature's way of healing the losses that are inevitable in any life. Illness is loss, too—it can mean loss of body parts, mobility, energy, favorite activities, earning power, an entire way of life. Like Queen Innana, we need to provide ourselves with mourners to release us from the prison of the underworld that unresolved grief represents.

All loss needs our attentive grief—not only the loss of persons we love, or a pet, but losses of opportunity and fulfillment. If ill health has taken from you some cherished dream, that, too, must be honored with grieving. You have the right and the need to grieve that loss in order to put it behind you and see that it was a necessary part of your path. This is often difficult to do, but if we accept our lives as purposeful, and I think we have no choice but to do so, then our losses—no matter how painful at the time—are part of the Master Plan for our life. We do not need to carry the pain forever: we have been given the healing power of grief. Here are some affirmations you can use.

I allow my grief for ( ) to flow naturally.
The grief I feel is part of my healing process.
Grief is nature's way of restoring me to balance.

The Grieving Process

When you have suffered a loss, no matter how major or how minor, there are five stages you must go through to utilize the healing power of grief:

1. Angst
2. Anger
3. Analysis
4. Acceptance
5. Action

Compare these five phases to the fingers of your hand. Each has a separate function, but together they operate as a unit. And just as you'd find your normal daily activities impaired if you burned your thumb or cut your pinky, you'll have to suffer through the emotional disruption of your life as you go through all these phases, consecutively and completely, before you'll be able to return to your normal functioning self.

Angst, the German word for pain, has come to mean that mental anguish we call *despair*. It is the first, and in some ways the most important, step of the healing process. Oddly enough, many people do not allow themselves to feel their pain—not even when a loved one dies. ("I have no time for tears.") In our society, both the bereaved and the ill are encouraged to "buck up" and repress or deny their feelings of grief, and those who do not impose their grief on others are much appreciated by their friends and relations. ("She's taking it so well!") Thus the cleansing and healing emotion is denied. Acknowledging your right to the pain is the first step.

Admitting your *anger* is next. The unfairness of it all! Let out those feelings of hate and frustration. Don't feel guilty about your rightful anger. Get fighting mad and yell your head off if you like. Say all those frightening and wounded feelings out loud. Hit a pillow or pound the bed. We are talking about *healthy anger* appropriately expressed and then let go.

It is often extremely difficult for a bereaved person to express anger toward the deceased. To openly acknowledge such feelings seems like a betrayal of love. As I progressed through the stages of grief for the loss of my mother, I came to realize that my father had not been able to express his overwhelming anger at his beloved wife for leaving him, nor at his God for allowing her to die. His unreleased anger had fermented into a poisonous resentment of me for being alive. Unexpressed anger leads to a sense of helplessness, which is associated with illnesses as varied as ulcers, heart disease, and cancer.

The next step is *analysis*. Do you really feel as helpless and bereft as you think you do? Examine your options. Is it that you really *can't* manage or that you are choosing not to do so? Has there been damage to your self-image or self-confidence? Examine your own responsibility in the matter, not with any feelings of guilt, but for the purpose of *taking control*. Once we can see clearly how we ourselves are involved in any situation, it becomes much easier to wrestle the demon down.

Once you have accomplished the above, you are ready to *accept* the facts of the situation, and then begin to see how you can change them. Clear out the emotional remains of the day and look for the lesson. Every cloud does have a silver lining.

The end of the process is *action*—becoming involved in your treatment and recovery. A study done at UCLA found that patients who developed an active way of coping with their stress were significantly more likely to remain free of disease than those who remained passive. This has been called the "fighting spirit."

The Healing Power of Release

Fear and resentment are twin demons of the psyche—what we fear, we resent. Resentment is anger held back. Both are major stressors. Resentment can produce gallstones. ("What she is doing really galls me.") It can also produce cancer, when what's eating *at* you starts eating *you*. Self-hate is a product of resentment, for being unable to vent our feelings makes us feel powerless. Taught to despise weakness, we turn the hate on ourselves, with deleterious results.

At the onset of World War II, President Franklin D. Roosevelt said, "We have nothing to fear but fear itself." Honoring this, America, in its darkest hour, was galvanized to slough off its former isolation; mobilize its considerable resources, both human and material; and, as ultimate victor, emerge on the world stage as undisputed leader.

The irony of fear is that what we fear rarely happens, but fear keeps our endocrine systems on red alert. By constantly activating our fears, we weaken our system by calling up the "fight or flight" mode as if *we are preparing for disaster*. By anticipating the worst, we set into motion the creation of a self-fulfilling prophecy. The way to turn this around is to release the fear the minute it rears its ugly head. Recognize it for what it is—a phantom—and send it back to the universe to be transmuted into positive energy. Bless your fears, for sometimes they can be genuine warnings. Examine them for information you can use, and then release them. Here are some affirmations you can use to release fear.

All my fears are now dissolved in universal goodness.
I loose this fear and let it go, expecting only good.
Recognizing that fear has no power, I now release fear.

Creating Your Place of No Fear

Deep within everyone is a place of no fear. When you emerged into this world from your mother's womb, you did not fear life but welcomed it. Soon thereafter, however, the adults around you began to instill fear in you. Admonitions such as "Don't do that, you'll get hurt," "Be careful," "Watch out, you'll fall down," became your childhood litany. Soon, what was a healthy ability to face life's challenges became fear—fear of coming to harm, fear of failure, fear of rejection, fear of loss. The list is long, and no doubt you know it well. Here is a meditation I created to assist my clients in overcoming their fears of all kinds.

Find a time when you can be alone and undisturbed for at least half an hour. Create an atmosphere of absolute calm around you. Light a candle, play soft music, scent the air—whatever gives you a sense of serenity and peace. Make sure your clothing is loose and comfortable, then breathe deeply and exhale all negative feelings and fears.

Now, create in your imagination a lovely place where you can feel totally safe and free from all fear. It might be a secluded spot in the woods, or a cove on a deserted beach. This place is your sanctuary. As this picture emerges within you, let yourself be absorbed into its quiet, beauty, and sense of safety.

When you have created a feeling-toned picture, fill in all the details. Imagine the colors, smells, textures, and sounds that such a place would have. Make this picture as complete as you possibly can. Remind yourself that no fear or threat can ever enter this space. Feel its protective vibrations.

When you feel totally comfortable in this space and have succeeded in creating a sense of safety here, look around and fix all the details in your memory. This is a place you can go whenever fear strikes to banish it from your psyche.

Now, slowly breathe yourself back to normal waking consciousness and notice how refreshed you feel when you realize that you have nothing to fear but fear itself.

Resentment can lead to the desire for vengeance. So long as you are involved with resentment, you are controlled by it, which

The Healing Mind

wastes vital energy. Mired in the past, you cannot move freely into your future. Releasing resentment has nothing to do with the other person—*do it for yourself.* Here are some affirmations you can use for resentment.

> *I now reclaim my own power in this situation.*
> *I release all that is not positive for my life.*
> *What happened in the past is now over and done with.*
> *My love for myself overcomes all resentment.*

Resentment Neutralizing Exercise

To do this meditation, first use breathing and relaxation techniques. When you feel ready, allow yourself to sink into a deep state of relaxed consciousness. Tell your SELF that you are now ready to let go of all resentments.

Imagine a bubble of beautiful royal purple drawing up in front of you like a magical carriage. Step inside. There find an altar on which is a flame of purple fire. Speak your resentment to the flame, which will consume it.

Next, see a pool of purple-tinted water, and allow all resentments to come to its surface. Transfer them one by one to the purple flame, and watch them go up in lavender smoke.

Finally, when the water in the pool is clear of all your resentments, wash your hands in it and proclaim, "I am now free of all resentment. I now release all resentment forever."

Let the purple flame flare up, burning higher and higher until its peak has reached your Higher Self. Give thanks and slowly allow yourself to return to consciousness.

Healing Mind, Body, Spirit

The Healing Power of Forgiveness

Odd as it may seem, the act of *forgiving* has immense healing power. When we carry within us—encoded into our flesh and bones—hate, anger, grudges, and other negative feelings about ourselves and others, we weaken our own immune systems and open ourselves to becoming ill. It has been said that hate kills. Not only does it kill others, as in the case of assault, murder, or genocide, but it kills ourselves as well. But how is one to forgive heinous crimes, or even lesser incursions, that have caused us to suffer psychological and/or bodily injury?

The secret is that *to forgive* does *not* mean *to approve*. Nor does it mean that we are to welcome the perpetrator back into our affections and regard. It only means that we must *let go within ourselves* of the negative emotions that are poisoning our systems. If we hate and resent—no matter how justified these feelings are—we do the most harm to ourselves. Unless we act out in a violent way, the hated person suffers far less than we do. Hate acts like a corrosive on both spirit and body, a contaminant that flows through our cells like acid, burning everything it touches. To paraphrase, the road to health is paved with forgiving intentions.

When I first learned of the healing power of forgiveness, I was most skeptical. My anger and hate had previously served me as a source of strength and even survival during some pretty tough times. It got me going when there was no discernible reason for continuing on. Like many protective devices erected in childhood to defend against the onslaught of conditions over which the child has no control, mine had worked for a time, when crisis was a way of life.

But, like all defensive constructions, those emotions of hate and anger began to strangle me once they had served their survival purpose. I had used them when I had no other defenses, but they had outlived their usefulness and were becoming deleterious. I recognized it was time to let them go. And letting go is what forgiveness is all about—flushing that corrosive acid out of *your* system, for *your* own purposes, to help *yourself*. It's not about the other person. It's about *you* and *your* health and happiness.

Despite feeling downright silly doing it—for one thing, a lot of these people were dead—I began to practice forgiveness, consciously calling to mind those for whom I felt enmity. Catharine Ponder advises making a list of all those who need your forgiveness. My list was long, and it grew longer as I remembered many experiences I had tried to forget. I was sure I had embarked upon a hopeless endeavor. Still, I persisted, sitting for thirty minutes each day and mentally forgiving everyone who had ever hurt me.

Some were easier to forgive than others. My father was, of course, the most difficult. Though I had had no contact with him for ten years, he remained alive and horrible in my psyche until my consistent practice of forgiveness bore the fruit of cleansing and healing. So, even if you think you can't possibly forgive those who have harmed you grievously, keep at it for your own sake. At first, the practice of forgiveness can reactivate bad feelings, reopen old wounds. However, these psychic and emotional poisons we ingested as children, and later on as well, need to be flushed out of our systems to prevent them from doing serious damage to our health. Forgiveness lets old wounds be cleaned out and finally healed. Look at it this way: if you accidentally ingested a poisonous substance, you wouldn't hesitate to stick your finger down your throat in order to get it out of your system, even if that's an unpleasant activity.

As I went down my list of those who had abandoned me, betrayed me, not been there for me when they should have been, withheld love, robbed me of my childhood and my heritage—a long and dreary recounting—mentally forgiving them all one by one, some very interesting things began to happen.

☙ *Healing Mind, Body, Spirit*

Inside, old tensions loosened and relaxed; self-destructive behaviors or ones I didn't like were easier to control, or forgo. Most interestingly, several weeks into my daily forgiveness meditations I realized that—after years of suffering bouts of serious and debilitating flu annually or more often if I was stressed—an entire winter had passed without my once having the flu or even a cold.

Forgiveness has the ability to reach deep into the implicate order of your SELF and heal long-standing, chronic conditions. You don't have to believe it to try it. Practicing forgiveness is risk-free. You have nothing to lose and everything to heal.

Put yourself on your forgiveness list, too. Mentally forgive yourself for anything you feel needs forgiving. The wearing of the hair shirt of guilt is not conducive to healing. Here are some affirmations you can use.

> *I invoke the healing power of forgiveness.*
> *I forgive everybody and everything that has hurt me.*
> *Forgiveness cleanses my cells and brings me healing.*

How to Practice Forgiveness

Your "forgiveness ritual" can be very simple. The great healers of Hawaii, the Kahunas, knew healing principles we are now rediscovering. They practiced "burning the rubbish in the mind" techniques to cleanse the mind of guilt and hate, whatever was "eating up inside" the patient being treated.

You can use the method described previously: set aside half an hour each day, sit quietly, and mentally forgive everyone you can think of who has ever hurt or harmed you in any way whatsoever. Start with the lesser and more recent experiences—the small hurts and stings that nonetheless can be painful. (There is an old saying, "We can sit on a mountain but not a tack.") Perhaps you were snubbed by someone, unfairly criticized by a friend, fired from a job. Begin along these lines and work your way back to the most painful and deep-seated traumas of your life. One by one, like counting beads on a string, forgive each person and tick off the name.

Forgiving need not involve the other person in any way. This is a private matter, your own personal housecleaning. It involves only the letting go of bad feelings resulting from past experience. And if you happen to encounter someone who was on your list, you will be pleasantly surprised to discover that your reaction to that person will be different than before. Not only that, but as you change your attitudes toward others, they will automatically respond by altering their attitude toward you.

The Healing Power of Acceptance

It may seem strange, but *acceptance* is a powerful tool in your personal first-aid kit. By acceptance I most emphatically do not mean *resignation*. Acceptance carries with it the possibility of saying, "No." When you are able to accept the circumstances life deals you, you are then in a position to make changes. As the neurolinguists like to say, "When life hands you a lemon, make lemonade." In other words, accept what *is* and then begin to reprogram to make the changes you want. Here are some affirmations you can use.

I accept this condition for the purpose of changing it.
I can change whatever I choose to change.
This situation has been given to me for a purpose.

Acceptance Meditation

To do this exercise, find a comfortable position and begin by taking several deep breaths to relax yourself completely. Close your eyes and imagine yourself standing before a mirror that has the power to show you your true self—not just your physical reflection, but a reflection of your innermost reality. Look carefully at this reflection and examine what you see. *Do not make judgments.* Do not criticize yourself. Do not turn away. Do not be squeamish or embarrassed. Just look.

Now, while looking at this reflection of your true self, say softly and gently in your mind, "I accept you. I truly accept you for who you are and who you can be. I accept all of you. I accept that you are a true reflection of my SELF. I know that by accepting you I can make any changes that I want or choose."

Repeat this several times until you feel that you are speaking the truth to yourself, that you are genuinely able to accept yourself with all your pain and shortcomings, but also with all your wonderful potential to heal and grow.

Now, slowly breathe yourself back to normal consciousness and give thanks for the ability to accept.

The Healing Power of Words

The healing power of words is immense and not to be underestimated. It is the very cornerstone of the healing methods of "practical Christianity," as practiced by the Unity Church, the Church of Religious Science, and others.

The Healing Mind

Myrtle Fillmore, with her husband Charles, founded Unity Church. Kansas City-born, she had previously been a schoolteacher, a wife, and a mother, worshipping as a Methodist and leading a traditional life.

The year 1886 brought a startling change into her life. She was diagnosed with tuberculosis, at the time considered incurable. Doctors gave her six months to live. Though the Fillmores were conventional people, their desperate situation opened them up to exploring paths other than the ones offered by Mrs. Fillmore's doctors. They attended a metaphysical lecture on healing and there heard the words, "You are a child of God, therefore you do not inherit sickness." These words made a great impact on the sick woman, who believed her TB was an inherited condition about which she could do nothing except wait to die. Here is her own account of how she healed herself through the power of words, as reported by James Dillet Freeman in *The Household of Faith*:

> I have made what seems to me a discovery. I was fearfully sick; I had all the ills of mind and body that I could bear. Medicine and doctors ceased to give me relief, and I was in despair when I found practical Christianity. I took it up and I was healed. I did most of the healing myself, because I wanted the understanding for future use. This is how I made what I call my discovery.
>
> I was thinking about life. Life is everywhere—in nature and in man. "Then why does not the life in the worm make a body like a man's" I asked. Then I thought, "The worm has not as much sense as a man." Ah! Intelligence, as well as life, is needed to make a body. Here is the key to my discovery. Life has to [be] guided by intelligence in making all forms. The same law works in my own body.
>
> Life is simply a form of energy, and has to be guided and directed in man's body by his intelligence. How do we

communicate with intelligence? By thinking and talking, of course. Then it flashed upon me that I might talk to the life in every part of my body and have it do just what I wanted. I began to teach my body and got marvelous results.

I told the life [in my organs] that it was...active and strong. I went to all the life centers in my body and spoke words of Truth to them—words of strength and power. I asked their forgiveness for the foolish, ignorant course that I had pursued in the past, when I had condemned them and called them weak, inefficient, and diseased. I did not become discouraged at their being slow to wake up, but kept right on, both silently and aloud, declaring words of Truth, until the organs responded.

After her remarkable recovery, as Unity's cofounder she went on to become a noted spiritual healer and lived for another forty years.

What is astonishing to me about this passage, written more than one hundred years ago, is that in it are adumbrated the morphic field theory of Sheldrake, the "information universe" theory of Foster, and the quantum physics of the new scientific paradigm. Myrtle Fillmore experienced what our present-day scientists are only beginning to understand: that the universe is filled with intelligence and that our human bodies, as part and parcel of the universal plan, are likewise filled with radiant intelligence, which responds to our communicating with it.

While I do not contend that affirmations alone can alter the course of serious illness or disease—all of these healing powers should be used in tandem—my personal experience has taught me of the sheer POWER in words, both positive and negative.

Words can be sharpened into rapier-sharp points that stab deep and leave lasting wounds. They can become shrapnel, exploding in our psyches and penetrating to the very marrow of our bones and beings.

The Healing Mind

Or, words can be lullabies, soft comforters, soothing tonics, and healing vessels. Use them wisely and with care, for each word you utter, to yourself or to others, is powerful. A single word can change a life, for better or for worse. One of the most often used words that produces terrible impact is *stupid!* Children labeled with this epithet may never learn. Their "learning disorder" has nothing to do with brain acuity and everything to do with what they believe to be the truth about themselves.

Enid Hoffman, an expert on the Hawaiian Kahuna, says that the oral cavity is a resonating chamber in which words, silent or sounded, reverberate in specific vibrational patterns in the brain. In the same vein, moaning and groaning about your mental, emotional, and physical ills will make them worse, not better. Martyrs are always on their way to the death chamber, in one way or another. So, watch your words as closely as you would watch the possession and use of a gun. Don't pull the trigger without first thinking about what you are saying, and why. Here are some affirmations that you can use.

My SELF knows what is best for me, knows how to heal.
I give thanks for the healing power in my every cell.
My life force strengthens and renews me daily.

Affirmative Meditation

To do this meditation, first use breathing and relaxation techniques. When you feel ready, allow yourself to sink into a deep state of relaxed consciousness. Tell your SELF, "My powers of healing are unlimited. I acknowledge that I can be healed. I am being healed now. All imbalances in my mind, body, emotions, and spirit are being adjusted back to their original perfection. I know that healing is possible because all things are possible to my unlimited SELF. I am being transformed within and without. I am in harmony with my own deep purpose of being. I am being relieved of all impediments to living my life fully and in perfect health. I now proceed with my life in a new spirit of faith, courage, and happiness. I release and let go of all pain, illness, and disease and return them to the universal source for transformation into positive healing energy. I give thanks for the lessons learned through my difficulties, and I heal myself of any negative effects."

You can also use the healing power of words by writing them down. Spending a few minutes each day writing affirmations to apply to a specific condition can be a helpful exercise. The ancient Chinese believed so strongly that words were power sources that anything written was preserved for all time. A favorite technique of mine is to write on a piece of paper all negative conditions that need to be removed and then burn the paper. It is said that the energy of fire purges.

Words can be sung or chanted. In India, a country with a rich tradition of spiritual healing, it is thought that words that are sung are the most powerful of all words. You can make songs of your affirmative statements. I like to put mine into "rap" form, a syncopated sound that doesn't require any singing talent. Whichever way you choose to manifest your words—by thinking silently, speaking, writing, singing—choose them with utmost care and acknowledge their power.

The Healing Power of Images

The marvelous mechanism of the mind can do almost anything: it can make you sick, but it can also make you well. A unique

The Healing Mind

characteristic of our minds is their *power to make images*. Symbolic images arise from the deepest unconscious levels of our beings and carry with them great power to affect our emotions and bodies. Imaging seems to switch on an inner power that works to produce the imagined result: the thought-image sinks deep into the subconscious and works upward into life.

Our ability to program—or reprogram—our deep inner minds with images during the alpha-theta, or self-hypnotic, state connects our conscious minds with our unconscious—the explicate with the implicate orders because the creative, right brain thinks in images. The healing power of images can help us to manifest the conditions we desire in our lives.

The healing power of images is well known in the psychoimmunology field. The many instances of the use of imagery—to relieve pain, to bring disease into remission, to slow the rate of increase in various illnesses—have been well documented. This is called *therapeutic imagery* and it is practiced in stress and pain clinics, cancer treatment centers, and other medical venues. You do not, however, have to attend a clinic to use the healing power of images. You can do it right now in the privacy of your own home.

Researchers have found that the use of self-guided, directed imagery can change the very cells of our bodies, in some instances almost instantaneously. Your mind is the programmer for your body, not the other way around, and visualizations reach into the deepest levels of your being.

Also, placebo experiments have proved that you have the power to heal yourself because the body does not know the difference between what is "real" and what is imagined. It acts on imagined information just as effectively, or more so, than on sensory information coming in from the outside environment. So, if you *act* as if something were true, *voila*! Sooner or later it comes true. This is because visualizations set up a *neurological template*, which is a blueprint or program of instructions for the

Healing Mind, Body, Spirit

body to follow. You can both *program* and *deprogram* yourself. You can change negative patterns and belief systems.

Psychologists Georgia Nigro and Ulric Neisser of Cornell University were interested in discovering which methods of visualization worked best. They organized three groups of people to play darts. The first group was told not to practice. The second group was instructed to visualize themselves throwing the darts just as if they were doing it. The third group made a mind movie of themselves throwing the darts at the board and watched it. Then they stepped into the movie and did it. Not surprisingly, the group that did not practice at all scored lowest. What was surprising was that the third group showed *twice* the accuracy as the second group.

Before you begin your visualizations, set up a private screening room in your imagination, just like a movie mogul has in his mansion. Yours, however, is the mansion of the mind, a far vaster domain than a mere physical structure.

To do this, set up a mental screen, like a TV or a film screen, on which you will view your mind movies. Here are some affirmations you can use.

I now create powerful, healing images for myself.
The images I make have the power to heal me totally.
My images are my medicine and will cure me.

How to Make Mind Movies

The key to the healing power of images is *to envision yourself as already being in the desired state*. Next, fill your movie with rich sensory details. Your subconscious mind responds to information about the realm of the senses. Imagine *being* the person you really want to be. *See, hear, and feel* what that would be like. "Put on" that person, so to speak, like you would put on a beautiful coat. Walk around in your ideal self, feeling down to your toes and bones what that experience would be like. How does it feel?

Remember, this is *your* movie. You are the writer, producer, director, *and* the star. You don't need to worry about the *how* of it; that will take care of itself. You only need to richly imagine the end result and see yourself as having attained it.

A clear mental picture of the goal and the circumstances that will surround it is the path to success. Vague wishes or unspecific thoughts won't work. Don't say, "I wish I felt better," and try to turn that thought into a mind movie. Instead, think "I want to be fit, energetic, totally free of all aches and pains," and then see yourself as you would be in that desired state. Maybe you are playing ball on the beach, full of energy and able to run and jump. Perhaps you are throwing away your pills because you don't need them anymore. The specific images are up to you. It's essential that the images you choose have *meaning* for you.

When you have created your perfect picture of health, and whatever else goes along with it, run your mind movie on a screen that you have set up for it. If you like, stage it as a play. You are going to watch your mind movie three times, in progressive sequences. The first time, just run it through and watch closely to see what you can refine or improve, like a rehearsal or trying on clothes to see if they fit right. At this point, you are critiquing, not participating. The second time is a dress rehearsal with all of the details in exact place, just as it will be on opening night. There's even an audience—you—to applaud your efforts. On the third viewing, *you see yourself actually stepping into the role you have designed for yourself.* This is the real thing and you are *in it*, not just observing or critiquing.

Healing Mind, Body, Spirit

The treasure-map technique that follows is an excellent adjunct to visualizations, especially for those who may find it difficult to conjure up pictures in the mind. By using actual pictures that symbolize what you want to achieve, you produce the desired effect.

Treasure-Map Technique

To make a "treasure map," you'll need a large piece of poster board, glue or tape, and pictures. You can cut pictures from magazines of healthy-looking people doing things you would like to be able to do. When you have collected a sufficient number of pictures representing your wishes, paste them on the poster board in any manner that appeals to you, using an image of particular significance at the center. Some people like to use a religious symbol; some use a photograph of themselves. Once you have made your treasure map, put it where you can view it often. Spend a few minutes viewing it in a relaxed state just before sleep, and again just after waking. You can also make a portable treasure map by using a small notebook, which you can flip through during free moments away from home.

chapter eight
The Healing Spirit

Much illness may have its roots in unrecognized spiritual distress—issues of isolation, of anger, the feelings people have that they don't matter or that nobody matters to them.... There is a general lack of meaning and purpose and significance that seems to underlie illness. What we call stress might really be spiritual isolation. It might really be an insensitivity to and a lack of recognition of our spiritual needs. And so they are unmet because they are unrecognized—and we are spiritually isolated.

                     ∽ Rachel Naomi Remen, M.D.
                                 Noetic Sciences Review

Healing Mind, Body, Spirit

Since time began, people have dealt with the profound issues of pain, illness, and healing in essentially spiritual ways, from the elaborate rituals of the Babylonians, Egyptians, and Mezzo-American cultures to the dream-inducing methods of the ancient Greeks. Ours is the only culture in history with a medical system that does not recognize a spiritual component in the healing process, nor make any attempt to invoke its power.

The impact of spiritual factors on health is difficult if not impossible to measure scientifically. However, the widespread interest, use, and belief in spiritual practices for healing, as well as for maintaining good health, is a prime untapped area for research and clinical application. It is like an undiscovered gold mine, just waiting for its riches to be brought to the surface.

The relationship of the spiritual approach to healing is controversial—and the issues involved in studying it are complex. Medical training in Western society does not equip the physician to deal with the spiritual dimensions of healing. Most scientifically trained practitioners shy away from any contact with spirituality, which they consider to be unscientific. Yet, cultures throughout history have had a spiritual base to their healing rituals, practicing what might be termed "spiritual technology." In these traditions, mental and physical distress alike are seen to be linked to spiritual disorder, sometimes called "soul loss," which refers to damage done to the essential, inviolate core—the essence of the person's being. Injury to this vital center can manifest as immunological impairment, cancer, severe depression, and other serious conditions.

Spiritual practice of whatever kind aims to balance the person—or to rebalance when difficulties arise—through communication with a higher power. *Intentionality* is a key—we seek to alter or uplift ourselves or our conditions, including health, through some form of spiritual communion.

The Healing Spirit

The form itself is irrelevant—all roads at the bottom of a mountain lead to the summit. The question is not one of *how* we arrive at a spiritual dimension to our lives, and to our healing process, but one of admitting the possibility into our consciousness.

Today increasing interest in the connection between spirituality and healing is indicated by the strong upsurge of media attention this topic is receiving. Articles in major mainstream publications, such as *American Health*, the *Wall Street Journal*, the *New York Times Magazine*, and even the *Journal of the American Medical Association*, ask provocatively, "Should physicians write 'prayer'…when prescribing for their patients?" Prayer is, of course, only one form of spiritual observance. On December 6, 1995, the *Christian Science Monitor* ran the headline "The Healing Role of Spirituality Gains Ground."

At the same time this article appeared, a conference entitled "Spirituality and Medicine" was held under the auspices of Harvard Medical School to bring together medical personnel and religious advisors. And, the National Institute for Healthcare Research has sponsored a conference on "Spiritual Interventions in Clinical Practice."

How does a spiritual focus help to heal? First, people who have a deep conviction and belief in a transcendent reality are better able to disconnect from the idea that the body and its ails are "all there is." By connecting to a higher power—however one experiences this or chooses to define it—we bring forth our inner sense of innate wholeness. We are able to see ourselves as *spiritually perfect*, even when suffering ill health. This promotes our ability to reconnect with our implicate patterns of health.

One study, *The Faith Factor*, sponsored by the John Templeton Foundation, found that spiritual factors are associated with increased survival and a reduction of anxiety, depression, and anger; reduced blood pressure; and improved quality of life for patients with cancer and heart disease. On average, it was found across the board—throughout different ages, ethnicities, religions, diseases, and conditions—that spiritual commitment produces a lifetime of health benefits. Says Dr. Herbert Benson in *Timeless Healing*, "Perhaps instinctively human beings have always known that worshipping a higher power was good for them. It could be a survival instinct."

In the many documented cases of "spontaneous remission" on record, some patients have said that spiritual communion played a significant role in their recovery by giving them a renewed sense of purpose in their lives.

The Healing Power of Prayer

Prayer has been shown to heal. In a well-known experiment by cardiologist Randolph Byrd of San Francisco General Hospital, people from across the country were asked to pray for approximately half of the nearly four hundred patients in coronary care. This was what is called a "double-blind" or controlled experiment in which no one involved, except the researchers, knew who was being prayed for and who was not. The prayed-for group did better on several counts. The death level was lower, they did not require life-support systems, and they needed much less medicine.

Research has also shown that it doesn't matter what the person's religious belief is in order for the healing to work. Even nonbelievers can be effective prayers. Though avid religionists, such as born-again Christians, test well, so do Buddhists—for whom Buddha is not a god but an enlightened human being. Even agnostics can pray successfully. Many "nondenominational" groups, such as Unity, use prayer as part of regular healing services, as do "spiritual" churches that practice prayer healing.

Prayer seems to work from some deep well of humanity's ability to feel compassion and empathy for those in need. It is the same impulse that acts when a person risks life and limb in an emergency situation to rescue a stranger from peril. Prayer need not be in the format or context of any formalized ritual or organized church.

How and *why* does prayer work to heal—or to do anything else, for that matter? Prayer aligns us with the cosmos, with the right and natural order of all things, or so I believe. When we pray for ourselves or others, we are putting ourselves into alignment with universal forces. One might say that we are deliberately getting in tune with the harmonic chords of the universe. And when we are in tune, we produce effects.

Cambridge biologist Rupert Sheldrake, author of *A New Science of Life*, has proposed a fascinating hypothesis that provides a possible explanation for prayer's effectiveness. The type of prayer known as "distant healing" suggests the "morphogenetic fields" Sheldrake's theory advances.

According to Sheldrake, these immaterial fields are unbounded by space and time. They contain a feedback loop in which the field structures the matter within it and in which the qualities of the matter modify the field. All organisms are seen as dynamic structures continuously re-creating themselves under the influence of their own past states.

A key concept here is that *matter and energy cannot be separated*. The fields surrounding matter are basic to understanding the phenomena within these fields, including not only the field for you and for me but those larger fields of the physical universe, all the way into the farthest reaches of space. New kinds of fields, both biological and consciousness-related, are being proposed, based upon the idea that the universe works like a hologram, in which every part interpenetrates every other part, thereby transmitting any change to the whole. Our brains, too, are holograms that construct "reality" by interpreting frequencies from a dimension transcending time and space. Thus, each of us can be considered to be a portion of the original Universal

Hologram, which in some sense created us and everything else in the universe according to its holistic pattern. Prayer lines us up with this pattern, in ourselves and in the universe. As we resonate with the universal pattern, we influence our personal pattern.

Prayer is also a form of meditation. It puts us into an altered state of consciousness not unlike the ones used for self-hypnosis and visualization. When we pray, we are actually visualizing the result desired even if we are not doing that consciously. Claude Bristol in *The Magic of Believing*, says, in relation to the law of suggestion,

> [F]orces operating within its limits are capable of producing phenomenal results. That is, the power of your own suggestion starts the machinery into operation or causes the subconscious mind to begin its creative work [which] leads to belief, and once this belief becomes a deep conviction, things begin to happen.

Lewis Thomas, chancellor of the Sloan-Kettering Cancer Center in New York, holds the view that the mind can play a powerful role in combating an infectious disease—a view not generally shared by physicians. In discussing the dramatic case of an English boy severely disfigured by viral warts who was healed by hypnosis, Thomas commented that the warts responded positively because of an inner power we all have, "a kind of superintelligence," or an "inner controller." He believes that making contact with this force gives us the power to self-heal.

That we are all one is demonstrated by quantum physics—the science of the subatomic dimensions of the world. Recent experiments have proved that two electrons, having once been in contact but then separated—even by relatively immense distances—still have the effect of changing one another, immediately and to the same degree, without any energy exchanged or time elapsed. The implication is that somehow in some way the two electrons remain *united* through the fact that there once was contact.

Brian Josephson, Nobel laureate physicist of Cambridge University's Cavendish Laboratory, suggests that this phenomenon, known as "quantum nonlocality," may one day serve to explain puzzling effects such as the effectiveness of prayer at a distance. And Dr. Beverly Rubik of Temple University's Center for Frontier Sciences believes that what makes intercessory prayer work is the transfer of "information."

Physicist David Bohm suggests that "Meaning, which is simultaneously mental and physical, can serve as the link or bridge between realms," connecting mind and body. Prayer brings us to meaning, for in prayer we address what is meaningful. According to Bohm, mind, body, and meaning together express a whole. In this schema, mind and body are not two separate entities interacting like dance partners, but work as one indivisible entity, *in* and *through* one another.

In *Meaning and Medicine*, Larry Dossey, M.D., writes:

> Our illusions regarding the body—that it is mindless and purposeless, that it behaves essentially like a machine—have paved the way for the loss of meaning in health and illness. Yet for almost the entire history of civilization, meaning has been an essential part of healing. Even today, when *most* people on the face of the earth become ill, they are treated not in modern hospitals nor by physicians but by the folk healer, the shaman, the medicine man. For them, meaning is utterly essential in understanding their illness. Without knowing what a disease means, rational therapy cannot be chosen and "cure" is unthinkable.

When we pray, we are addressing this "ground from which the whole of existence emerges." There are many names for this ground of being—God, Buddha, the One, the All, Source, Spirit—and each of us addresses it in our own individual way.

Though in elucidating the powers of healing I have consistently given exercises or meditations appropriate to each, no one can tell you how to pray. Prayer is a private matter. I will, however, offer you a list of affirmations to be used in conjunction with your prayer, or to get you started praying if you don't already do so, and some meditative mind-prayers adapted from *Spiritual Mind Healing* by Ernest Holmes.

> *I am healthy, strong, peaceful, happy, and at rest.*
> *Spirit, which is active in me, flows throughout.*
> *I am well, buoyant, happy, free, and full of joy.*
> *My days are filled with energy, radiance, and health.*
> *My prayer now removes all obstacles to my healing.*
> *The purifying energy of Spirit moves through me.*
> *I give praise and thanksgiving for all blessings.*
> *I bless myself and all others.*
> *I invite the healing power of Spirit into my life.*

Spiritual Mind Prayers

Everything that I believe to be true about the Spirit, I understand is also true about myself. Its Goodness is my goodness. Its Power is my power. Its Presence in me is my true self. There is only one True Self.

Every day I believe I am receiving Divine Guidance and inspiration. I realize there is nothing in the universe opposed to me other than my own doubt or any negative force in my own mind. There is nothing that can hinder, impede, or impair my progress.

I shall remember at all times that it is Life that gives. I am its beneficiary. Quietness, confidence, and peace shall be mine. My every tomorrow will be better than today. I now accept that I have an Infinite Power at my disposal.

In Spirit, all is perfect. In Spirit I am perfect. Spirit is at the root of my being. I have an intimate Source from which I may draw strength and inspiration. This universal "I Am" finds expression through me as the individual "I." It is the very essence of my being and in it I realize my true nature.

Another way to include prayer in your healing process is to choose a focus word for your relaxation response exercises that is spiritually meaningful to *you*. Here are some commonly used terms that will help you to choose one for yourself.

Nondenominational Focus Words
ONE • ALL • SOURCE • SPIRIT • INFINITE

Christian Focus Words
FATHER • CHRIST • LORD • MARY • JESUS

Jewish Focus Words
SH'MA YISROEL • SHALOM • ECHOD

Islamic Focus Words
INSHA'ALLAH • MOHAMMED • PROPHET

Buddhist Focus Words
OM MANI PADMI HUM • OM

Hindu Focus Words
SHIVA • VISHNU • KRISHNA • BRAHMA

Goddess Focus Words
ALL MOTHER • ISIS • GODDESS • HATHOR • GAIA

Healing Mind, Body, Spirit

Here is a prayer I wrote, "To the Goddess."

> Our Mother, who art the Earth,
> Hallowed be Thy Name.
> The Queendom beneath our feet,
> Thy Will, its harmony.
> Blessed all Thy spaces,
> Sacred all Thy creatures.
> Give us this day our food and drink,
> And prevent us from Thy despoilation.
> Forgive us our trespasses against Thy holy body,
> And teach us to reverence Thee always.

Preparing a Sacred Space

Some people like to have a special place for prayer and meditation. To prepare a sacred space, choose where you want it to be. If you have the luxury of a separate room, that is ideal, but any space you can spare will do. It could be an alcove, a niche, or just a corner of a room you use regularly. The important thing is your intention to keep your space sacred. Though most people will want a space in their homes, your sacred space does not have to be indoors. For centuries people worshipped in the open—in grottos or caves, in groves of trees that were sacred to the goddess, or on mountaintops. Once you have chosen the space, mark it out mentally (or walk around it). With your arms outstretched, palms downward, say, "I now declare this space to be sacred."

Your sacred space can contain an altar if you like, and a chair or cushion. Some people mark out their sacred space by using a small rug to define the area. A table or shelf can serve as altar space on which you can put items of significance to you, such as pictures or photographs, one or more candles, crystals or other objects, a plant or fresh flowers. A container of water is thought to draw off negative spirits and must be emptied after

The Healing Spirit

each use and set out fresh every time you use the space. Native Americans "cleanse" the air by burning the herb sage. You can place a few leaves or a pinch of powdered sage in a shell or other flameproof dish and scent the air with its pleasant odor.

It's important to have a sense of reverence about your sacred space. Do not enter it unless you have properly prepared yourself. Do not permit others to enter it without your permission and the correct attitude. If you consistently treat it as *sacred*, it will become imbued with a sense of holiness.

Creating a Ritual

Today we have all but lost the sense of and use of ritual. Old forms have largely lost their meaning as we have become disconnected from them. The churchly rituals of childhood no longer serve any purpose in our modern lives. However, ritual is a way of connecting ourselves to the larger pattern, and we can successfully create our own rituals. Many people have already done this without quite knowing it—certain routines of their lives attain the importance of ritual, even becoming somewhat formalized, such as family gatherings that are marked by special food and drink and an order in which things occur. Children naturally both create and respond to ritual—such as that of getting ready for bed—and can be upset if the precise sequence isn't followed. "No, no. I get in bed *first* and *then* you bring Teddy Bear."

To create a ritual to use before entering your sacred space, you need only perform a few actions in a certain order. It could be something as simple as removing your shoes and outer clothing, washing your hands, and lighting the candles. Or it could be something more elaborate such as taking a bath in scented water, putting on a special garment reserved for the purpose (priests in all cultures have always worn ceremonial robes), arranging a few fresh flowers in the vase you always use, having a ceremonial drink of wine, tea, or water. Whatever actions you pick should represent what is meaningful to you. They should have the effect of making you feel you are entering your sacred space *within* in preparation to entering the sacred precinct without. In temples and shrines of old, there was an outer precinct through which one had to pass—often guarded by fierce-looking figures—in order to enter the inner holy of holies.

By performing a ritual and putting one's self in the right inner space, one readies for contact with the higher power. Once you enter your sacred space, you should have a form to follow. Perhaps you sit on your cushion or chair and breathe quietly for a few moments and then begin your prayer. I like to hold a large, smooth rose quartz crystal. As you work with creating ritual, you will find what suits you best. Feel free to make changes that seems appropriate until you find what resonates with your SELF.

The Healing Power of Thankfulness

Thankfulness is a form of prayer. We recognize this annually as Thanksgiving Day, originally a prayerful occasion rather than just a feast, and many people repeat a simple prayer of thanksgiving daily at meals.

When you are sick, being thankful for *anything* may seem a difficulty, but there is great healing power in gratitude. If you learn to practice "an attitude of gratitude" before any illness strikes, you will strengthen your immune system, which responds to all positive thoughts. And, if you do get sick, you can hasten your healing by thinking thoughts of thanksgiving.

No matter how bad a situation is, there is always something for which one can give thanks and feel grateful. When I was quite ill and bedridden with chronic fatigue syndrome and things seemed dark indeed, I searched for something to give thanks for. I was nestled comfortably in a mound of soft pillows and down quilts, and it occurred to me that the very bed which contained my sick body was something for which I could express gratitude. I did so, adding prayers of thanks for every little thing around me that served to ameliorate my discomfort, including the sweet little cat who loyally sat on my chest day and night for the weeks of my illness and recovery. The more thanks I gave, the better I felt.

When you give thanks, you are praising, and praising is a form of prayer. Many people go to their place of worship and offer prayers in a formal way and then come home and set about complaining and grumping about all sorts of things. If you are guilty of this transgression against good sense, begin now to praise and give thanks to all about you. Your words of thanksgiving will sink into your subconscious and do their healing work. Dr. Masaharu Taniguchi, a Japanese metaphysician who has had remarkable success in the healing of cancer, says in his book *You Can Heal Yourself*, "These ideas of…'Thank you' cure all diseases." Here are some affirmations you can use.

I give praise and thanksgiving for every good thing.
I give thanks for…(list everything you can think of).
Today I find many positive things to be thankful for.

Exercise in Thanksgiving

This is an easy exercise to do, and you should do it often. To do this, you need only get comfortable and relaxed. You can even do it while walking around or performing simple chores or errands.

Mentally go through all the rooms in your house, your work space, your property. Give thanks for each and every item or function you are glad you have available to you. Go into your kitchen and give thanks for your stove, refrigerator, the food in it, your dishes, cutlery, appliances, and conveniences. Tour your living room and the other rooms of your house or apartment and give thanks for the furniture, lamps, any appliances such as a TV, VCR, air conditioner—and for the electricity to run them. Do this for every room—give thanks for the clothes in your closets (even if you perpetually have "nothing to wear"), the linens on your bed, the rugs on your floors, every comfort and convenience you enjoy. Think of what you would miss especially if you did not have it, and give thanks specifically. So many of us take so much for granted until we find ourselves without the common amenities. Just having a roof over your head is deserving of your profound gratitude.

Then work through your garage and any outside property, giving thanks for your car (if you have one), lawnmower, and so on. Give thanks for your work space and whatever you have there, such as a computer, fax machine, telephone, comfortable chair, good lighting, even tape and paper clips. Next, turn to the people and animals that populate and benefit your life, and give thanks for them one by one.

Don't forget to praise your own personal attributes, from whatever you like about your looks to your skills and abilities. Be thankful you have a brain that can learn and solve problems for you, a heart that can give and receive love, a body that houses your SELF. Give praise to your bodily functions, for without those you would be miserable indeed! You will be amazed how long a list you can compile.

By the time you have finished this inventory, any aches and pains you were feeling will be less and you will have given your immune system a boost. Do this exercise every day, more often if you are under the weather. Once you have done it a few times, you will be intimately familiar with all you are grateful for, and you can take a shortcut. Simply say, "I give praise and thanksgiving for every good thing in my life."

~ The Healing Power of Love

What seems to make prayer effective for healing is genuine caring for the person for whom the prayers are being offered. Psychologist Lawrence LeShan, in *The Medium, the Mystic, and the Physicist*, says that for healing to happen, "It is essential that there be a deeply intense caring."

The Greeks recognized different forms of love: *eros*, the intensely personal feeling we have for someone with whom we are closely related, especially in a romantic or sexual way; *philia*, the generalized feeling of love we have for fellow humans; and *agape*, spiritual love. To this I add another category—*self-love*, which the elegant Greeks did not name, but which is essential for self-healing. Logically, if we are working to heal ourselves, we must love ourselves. This is easier said than done. In fact, psychiatrist M. Scott Peck flatly states in the bestselling *The Road Less Traveled* that

> The feeling of being valuable [i.e., worthy of love]...is a direct product of parental love. Such a conviction must be gained in childhood; it is extremely difficult to acquire it during adulthood....As a result of the experience of consistent parental love and caring throughout childhood, such fortunate children will enter adulthood not only with a deep internal sense of their own value but also with a deep internal sense of security....When these gifts have not been proffered by one's parents, it is possible to acquire them from other sources, but in that case the process of their acquisition is invariably an uphill struggle, often of lifelong duration and often unsuccessful.

That doesn't seem to offer much hope to those among us—a majority—whose parents fell short of Dr. Peck's standard, does it? However, I disagree with his pessimism on the grounds of personal experience. To my mind, where Peck goes wrong is in saying that a sense of worth and security must be acquired from "other sources," presumably outside one's self, for to be dependent upon the love of others is to fear loss of that love, court disaster, and be in danger of serious disappointment. The proper aim of the loving parent is to teach the child to love *itself.*

I would dispute Peck's theory that loved children always develop "a deep internal sense of their own value," because dependency in the love of another creates fear of the loss of that love, which engenders a sense of insecurity. In point of fact, self-love is the only kind you can ever count on. The love of others can grow cold, be withdrawn, have strings attached, or be snatched away by an unkind fate. But perfect love is possible: from you to your SELF. The love you generate and give to yourself is pure and inexhaustible, like the life force itself from which it emanates.

Peck suggests that the void can be filled by psychiatric counseling such as he practices. Unfortunately, a great deal of such therapy fails. Peck says,

> No matter how well credentialed and trained psychotherapists may be, if they cannot extend themselves through love to their patients, the results will be generally unsuccessful. Conversely, a totally uncredentialed and minimally trained lay therapist who exercises a great capacity to love will achieve psychotherapeutic results that equal those of the very best psychiatrists.

Certainly many of us, but especially women, have been taught and trained to regard ourselves as dispensable, even disposable. We are supposed to take care of the needs of others, giving out love and nourishment, while taking in little or nothing, receiving only lip service in return for depriving ourselves. Though the word *sacrifice* originally meant "to make sacred," it has come to mean forfeiting one's own legitimate needs in the service of attending the needs of others. This road-to-martyrdom style of life is about as far from sacred as one can get. It is ultimately destructive, not only for the person making the sacrifices but also for those for whom the sacrifices are made. There is a hidden price to be paid—always.

There is a telling tale from the real life story of Romain Gary, a former French ambassador and writer whose first book *A European Education* won France's most prestigious literary prize, the *prix Goncourt*. The Russian-born writer's mother was fiercely devoted to her only child, making sacrifices on a heroic scale, including depriving herself of food, to promote his welfare. As were many pre-revolutionary Russians, she was enamored of all things French, and when Gary was eight she declared that he would one day become a French ambassador. Thenceforth, she bent all her energies in this direction, literally *walking* from Russia to Paris with her young son in tow. The description of this journey is riveting.

When World War II began, Gary, as a French citizen, enlisted in the RAF and flew many dangerous missions. He was seriously wounded in a crash. But all during the time he was a fighter pilot, risking his life to free France from German occupation, and during his long and painful convalescence, he regularly received letters from his mother, written by hand. These letters were a lifeline for Gary, whose mother was more proud of France than de Gaulle himself. Without her constant encouragement, he says he would never have made it through the war and the injuries he received. However, when he finally returned home, he discovered that his mother had died more than two years previously! How was it that he kept getting her letters, those letters that kept him going through the darkest days of the war? The answer was simple.

Knowing that she was seriously ill and going to die soon, and realizing that her precious son would be in mortal danger constantly, this woman wrote hundreds of letters full of love and cheer, praising her son for his heroism on behalf of her beloved France. These she entrusted to a friend to mail to Gary each week. He was not to know his mother was dead until he was safely home from the war.

Such total devotion is amazing—but is it a good thing? In Gary's memoir of his mother, *Promise at Dawn*, he writes what I consider to be some of the most poignant words I have ever read. Gary had been married and divorced several times, never finding true happiness. After he recounts the litany of his mother's sacrifices and all-consuming devotion, he says, "And that is why I have spent my life dying of thirst beside so many beautiful fountains."

Experience has shown me that the sense of self-worth, the basis for self-love, can be had by recognizing that each of us is a SELF, a *Spiritually Evolving Life Force*, a work-in-progress so to speak. As such, you already *are* a worthy person—one who has a purpose for being on the planet—and you deserve love, no matter how your parents treated you or what wrong notions you absorbed in the past. Begin now to make corrections. The act of loving is a spiritual act, one of self-evolution. And as we contact our loving SELF, we come to recognize that self-love and love of others are woven from the same thread—that ultimately they are indistinguishable.

The secret that is revealed is that you already have all the love you need—the healing power of love—within you right now. Love is your birthright, and you don't have to wait for it to arrive via another person. You can give it to yourself. You can actually generate a flow of love by releasing it from within through your desire to give your SELF transforming love. Love can be produced deliberately just as thought can be produced on demand. We have only to turn on our "love spigot" and let it flow into us and then out into the world, from where it will return multiplied. A friend once quipped, "Cast your bread upon the waters and it will come back buttered."

The first step in generating the flow of love is to realize now that love is there within you and can be released into circulation through your thoughts, feelings, words, and actions. Once you have learned to generate love, you will never be short of it again. You will become free of the crippling demands of others, and you will never need to enter a relationship with anyone in order to receive love. Not only that, but once you have acquired the knack of generating love to yourself, you will see that the outer world responds in kind. Since you will have plenty of love—"to share and to spare"—others will feel loved by you and act accordingly. As you radiate love first to yourself and then outward to the world, every part of your life will begin to right itself—you will attract the right people, right situations, right conditions for your full health and happiness.

This love you can generate is *agape*, or divine love. You have only to call upon it and it is there for you to use. Do not wonder how love works, or where it comes from, but have the boldness to know you can release it from within yourself now and forever. It is a well that can never be empty. It does not depend on persons, places, or things. It is as free as the air you breathe, and just as necessary. I'd like everyone to know a wonderful truth—that when there is a need for love we can supply it from within ourselves, to ourselves (as well as to others). Begin now to speak words of love to yourself, especially to any afflicted part of yourself.

Wherever you are in your life, whatever problems you have now or have faced in the past, love is a powerhouse of healing energy. It connects you to all good in the universe, from which you can draw at will. Love has its origins in the spiritual meaning of life, not in the rat race of everydayness. When we love, we feel transported, as if into another dimension, and we truly are in a higher place. You can climb to the stars on a beam of love. Love can be your secret weapon with which you vanquish the sorrows and ills of life. Practicing generating love on a daily basis is like pouring out a healing balm over yourself. You will become quiet, peaceful, and filled with harmony. You will be in sync with your SELF. By becoming a constantly radiating center of love, by filling yourself with the love you carry within you, you heal what ails you and better your life in all ways. Here are some affirmations you can use.

I generate love from the inexhaustible supply that fills the universe.
Love flows through me at all times in proportion to my needs and desires.
The love within me is mine to have and to use for all good purpose.

How to Generate Love

You have the ability to generate love at will. To experience this, sit, recline, or lie down in a comfortable position and close your eyes. Begin with a breathing or relaxation response exercise. Picture your dominant hand in your mind. Find your hand mentally and begin sending it love. Radiate love out of your heart center to your hand. Soon it will begin to feel warm and alive. It is responding to the love you are generating. Now, send love to other parts of your body at will. Just concentrate on sending the love out, and feel it being received. Continue sending yourself love until you feel filled with a glowing warmth, emanating from your heart center. Picture this love as a beautiful, pure, white light cascading through your entire body, loosening tension, soothing emotional hurt, healing pain or discomfort. Say, "I give this total pure love to myself. I honor myself with love now." Feel this love energy pulsating through your entire being while you imagine it as a beam of light streaming out of your heart center and filling every cell in your body, every crevice in your emotions, every thought in your mind. See this beam of powerful, healing light leave your body and flow out to the universe, filling it with radiance. Now, see the radiance returning to you, entering your heart center, and filling you with even more love, connecting you to the meaning in yourself and the meaning in the universe.

If your inner self controls all physical functions, it also controls all *dysfunction*. While outside help can facilitate our healing, only we can make it happen. What follows is an exercise that will enable you to commune with your inner self through the body, its vehicle.

The goal of this technique is to reconnect our *whole* selves with the body, to reestablish that link we had with our physical selves when we first entered this earth plane and were separated from the umbilical cord, taking our first breath. We didn't hate ourselves then, and for quite a time thereafter we enjoyed exploring our bodies and, through them, our world. The aim is to dissolve bodily tensions, originating in lack of love, and free up our energies for healing and purposeful living.

Love Is a Many-Splendored Body

Choose a period of time—an hour or more—when you can be alone and undisturbed by others or outside distractions. First, take a warm bath scented with oil or salts. Gently wrap yourself in heated towels or a soft garment. Take a comfortable position reclining or supine. Close your eyes. Breathe several minutes, concentrating on the breath.

Focus your mind on your toes, sending them love. Feel your toes as living tissue and think of all they do for you. If images of imperfect toes arise in your mind, bless them and remind yourself that your toes are perfect in Spirit. Bask in the experience of your toes being alive and pulsing with the life-giving blood coming from your heart. Say to your toes, "I love you. I thank you for what you do for me. I promise in the future to treat you with love and respect."

Move to your feet, ankles, calves, thighs, hips, genitals, reproductive organs, and buttocks, repeating the exercise. As you do this, check to see if there is discomfort in any part of your body, and send it not only love but healing energy. As you proceed, repeat to each part of your body, "I love you. I thank you for what you do for me."

Continue upward, to your abdomen, chest, heart, lungs, shoulders, arms, hands. As you do this, experience a new feeling of aliveness in your body. Determine that you are going to be on intimate terms with your body, more intimate than the terms you have ever been on with another person.

Slowly, proceed to your throat, face, head, eyes, mouth, tongue, teeth, and scalp, giving love to each in turn, thanking them for what they do for you. You

> will be amazed at how much your body does for you all the time without being given a whit of praise. Love and praise yourself, part by part, and then see the whole of yourself as being in perfect health, residing in the perfect love you give yourself. Repeat this exercise frequently.

The Healing Power of Dreams

In his book *Meaning and Medicine*, Larry Dossey, M.D., says,

> One of the most significant possible breakthroughs in understanding how healing comes about is the realization that we all possess an inner source of healing and strength that operates behind the scenes with no help whatsoever from our conscious mind. This "secret helper" has not been given its due.

The writer-philosopher Aldous Huxley says, "this unknown quantity at once imminent and transcendent, at once physical and mental, at once subjective and objective...sustains me, preserves me, gives me a long succession of second chances."

I call this "secret helper" *the authentic self*. It is the implicate-order pattern, brought with us when we arrived in this world, which orders our lives from within. Like a ship's gyroscope, it works to stabilize us when we encounter life's rough seas. This inner authentic you is always there, intact, no matter what blows life delivers. You retain a memory of that you who you *are*. Our conscious mind contains that "factory installed" template and continually attempts to bring its design into being. Jung says the psyche strives for wholeness; illness is merely its way of correcting imbalance.

Healing Mind, Body, Spirit

A primary way in which the authentic self communicates with us is through dreams. People in many cultures, ancient and contemporary, have used dreams for healing. In the Greek temples of healing, the "god" was invoked through carefully induced dreaming. Native Americans used dreams for many purposes, one of which was to promote healing by contacting supernatural "spirits" who had the power to cure illness.

The first rule in using dreams for healing purposes is to take them seriously. People who regard their dreams as important and able to provide vital knowledge will both remember their dreams and receive information from them. While some psychotherapists regularly use dream interpretation as part of their treatment process, few in the medical profession have paid any attention to the healing power of dreams. Unfortunately, our society as a whole does not think dreams are of much use—I've never heard of a "dream support group." Therefore, it is up to the individual to honor and support his or her own dreaming process, to pay attention and heed information coming from the unconscious.

Here is a quite dramatic example of a healing dream I had recently in the wake of a major dilemma. After working for weeks to draft material for a new book on a topic close to my heart, I received a lukewarm response from the editor who previously had shown enthusiastic interest. She suggested major changes that distorted my original intention, but I nonetheless set to work on revising the material to her specifications. It was a grave mistake. In my eagerness to have my book published, I failed to notice that I broke one of my own commandments: *Be true to yourself at all costs*. Breaching my personal integrity by trying to please someone who, I woefully realized, was unable to understand the fundamental concept at the heart of the book, cost me dearly. The first symptom was the usual one: a sore throat. Instinct told me I was in trouble, and I took immediate preventive measures. However, the emotional and psychological damage had already been translated into my body—the piper was calling to be paid.

For two weeks, I was confined to my bed, coughing day and night while I worried about not getting the revision finished on schedule. Then, an ironic voice in my head advised, "If it's going to make you sick, don't do it!"

As I lay there in the third week of my suffering, utterly exhausted by the long bouts of coughing and the crushing ache my body had become, I dreamed of a wolf lying sick and alone on the forest floor, on a pile of dead leaves. Social animals, wolves live in packs, but this wolf had retreated to the forest to heal himself in isolation. He had nothing to help him but his innate wolf nature. His only course was to follow his deep instinctual knowledge of what would bring him back to health.

When I first saw him, he appeared to be unconscious—the sight of his limp, inert body with the glowing eyes filmed over brought a rush of compassion and love for him through me, and I desperately wanted to do something to help. As I stood over him, wishing I were a veterinarian, something magical happened—I *became* the wolf. And, as the wolf, I understood profoundly the meaning of *integrity*. In the human world, the word "integrity" has come to mean something like honesty, but what it really means is *wholeness*. What possesses integrity has never been compromised: it is in a state of completeness, undivided, unbroken. Though grievously ill, the wolf was in total possession of his integrity. He was, most deeply, *who he was*: absolutely true to his fundamental nature. He wasn't trying to please anyone or second-guess "the marketplace." He simply *was*.

Joseph Campbell says that "myth *is* metaphor"—not that something is *like* something else, but that it *is* the something else. I was not just dreaming about a wolf—I *was* the wolf! And, as the wolf, I lay there on the floor of the forest primeval and called up from within my wolf-self those most basic instinctive animal powers that sustain us *automatically*.

Healing Mind, Body, Spirit

My friend Stephen Larsen, professor of psychology, writes in *The Mythic Imagination*:

> [T]he novice shaman is shown *how important personal integrity is*....[T]he individual soul plunges into the depths of his or her own psyche in the search for renewed meaning...the shamanic journey has yielded transpersonal, and very reliable, maps...into the psyches of modern people in personal crisis....[A]n animal...may announce it.

Afterward, I slept for many hours, the first real sleep I'd had in the weeks of my illness. I woke feeling refreshed, clear-headed, and buoyant, as if I had been reborn. A vivid memory remained with me of actually *being* the wolf, a living creature with no one but Nature to call upon for healing. If you asked me to *consciously* pick an animal to be, one to represent my instinctual level of being, I'd have chosen a tiger or a dolphin. But the wolf-self was such a profound experience that I realized I had contacted my authentic self in animal form. Never shall I forget the sensation. Ever afterward I have been able to call it up at will. From this dream I gained a profound insight into my own inner workings, the importance to me of personal integrity, and the dangers inherent in my violating it. I decided to abandon the revision and stick to my vision, whatever the outcome.

In another vein, a female friend, who practices a hands-on healing therapy, related the following dream to me:

> I am working on a young man, an AIDS patient. I want so much to help him, but I know there is only so much I can do. Suddenly I see *myself* covered with the dark spots of the Karposi cancer. Thinking I have caught it from him, I step back in horror and begin frantically to try to peel the scabs from my body. I wake up shaken and tearful.

The Healing Spirit

This woman had devoted herself to treating AIDS patients and was utterly exhausted from the energy she was putting into them. She had already suffered from a weakened heart, but instead of taking the prescribed rest, she insisted on continuing her work, saying, "My patients need me." I had warned her about the risks of burnout and begged her to take a vacation, but she insisted on overextending herself "just this once." Repeatedly I admonished her to cut her patient load before she became sick herself, but, being a healer, she assumed she could heal herself if it came to that. Until she had this dream. Finally, she was able to understand the harm she was doing to herself in her efforts to do good for others, and to recognize the danger inherent in her selfless attitude. The dream vividly showed how her compulsion to "aid" was harming her. In this instance, the dream acted as a warning device, forcing her to acknowledge what she was ignoring. As Larsen says, "What seems to be called for…is the as-if metaphorical attitude that takes the dream and its implications symbolically and yet seriously."

A powerful example of this is a dream I had that explicated the resolution of one of my "simultaneous selves," as discussed in Chapter One. After I had made contact with my younger self and understood that I had to find a way to assimilate this "part self" into my mature whole being, I had the following healing dream, which I titled simply *Resolution*.

> I enter a room where a young woman is lying in bed, gravely ill. I do not know her. But as soon as she sees me she begins crying profusely, sobs wracking her body. I rush to her, climb into the bed with her, and take her tenderly into my arms, crooning to her and soothing her, as a mother would do with a child. Her sobs subside as she clings to me. Suddenly, she is quiet. She gazes at me intently as if recognizing me. I again fold her into my arms, embracing her with all of my self. We fall asleep locked together like lovers.

Healing Mind, Body, Spirit

You can activate and enrich your dream life by paying attention to it; by working on understanding your dream images every day; by keeping a dream diary; by discussing your dream experiences with others who dwell on their dreams; by asking for dreams to solve problems and promote healing generally, and specifically, by thanking your dream self for its help. Here are some dream affirmations you can use.

I trust my dreams to reveal to me my inner reality.
My dreams are gifts for which I give thanks.
My dreams are a form of self-therapy each night.

Finding Your Authentic Self

A technique that will enable you to contact the authentic Self within, one that you lost touch with and whose acknowledgment can bring you healing (and many other benefits) follows.

Get into a relaxed state and imagine yourself going for a walk in the woods. Look up at the tree limbs overhead, hear the birds singing and the burbling of a stream, smell the pine-scented air, feel the sun on your skin, drink in the atmosphere.

As you proceed along your walk, you are going to find a secret doorway—it might be in the trunk of a tree or buried in the ground. Maybe it is at the heart of a flower. When you find your secret door, open it and discover a passageway leading downward. Step in and begin to descend. It may be a stairway or a sloping path. As you go down, feel the magic of this place and know that you are entirely safe. This is going to be a great adventure. You are going to find your "original self," the one patterned in your implicate order, the one you were before parents and society laid their encrustations upon you, the one you *are* in perfect health, balance, and tranquility. As you descend and leave the upperworld behind, feel a sense of excitement, as if you were coming home after a long absence in foreign lands. At the bottom, you will find a lovely room, and there you will meet your authentic Self. When this Self appears, acknowledge him or her as being you at the best you can be, give thanks for this meeting, and return to the "real" world with the memory of who you truly are.

part four
The Cosmic Organism

chapter nine
The Transforming Crisis

Anyone seriously interested and willing to do a bit of systematic research can verify that the natal chart depicts the basic psychological and emotional makeup of the individual and...the potential developmental patterns likely to evolve.... Events occur in synchronistic conformity at such times as the field dynamics...resonate with the individual's readiness.

~ Edward C. Whitmont, M.D.
The Alchemy of Healing

Maladaptive behaviors resulting from childhood trauma and repressions that have become somatically ingrained in the very tissues of our bodies can be retrained to repair a damaged constitution, but we cannot change our fundamental nature. Basic patterns of who we *are* show clearly in the birth chart, making astrology a marvelous tool for fine-tuning ourselves to our already existing *a priori* implicate pattern. Since we have little or no control over who we find ourselves to be, it's important that we learn to accept ourselves. There is no amount of therapy, be it physical or psychological, that can change a fundamentally indrawn, shy person into an aggressive loud-mouth extrovert nor metamorphose a heavy-boned, driven personality into a fragile flower. We do not *create* who we are. At best, we *discover* it and use it well and wisely. For this reason, the exercises and meditations in this book are designed to connect you to who you already *are*. They are not intended to enable you to remake yourself in some idealized image.

Our native constitutions strive for homeostasis, or the status quo. We produce psychological immune reactions to ward off the invasion of what is new and disturbing. It is important to realize that "what is sauce for the goose is poison for the gander," and to recognize our reactions for what they are and honor how they affect us. These innate "psychological immune systems" cannot be simply disowned; they must be worked with in terms of one's own implicate pattern of personality and its current stage of development. To this end, we must examine how we operate on the explicate level, which we identify as body and mind, in order to come into meaningful contact with our implicate order, the internal compass by which we navigate the waters of life.

Astrology is a marvelous tool in this endeavor because it connects us to the cosmos, which possesses both intelligence and

The Transforming Crisis

purpose. Your birth was not an accident and your life is not a mere series of random events. You and the universe are One. You have the ability to decipher your part in the cosmic scheme, in order to get in tune with the plan for your life. As revealed by the study of astrology, the *natal* chart is calculated for the precise time and place of your birth, and works as an overall blueprint, while the timing of life crises, including those involving illness of both a physical and psychological nature, can be indicated by the *transits* of the planets in relation to the natal chart. (Transits are the daily movement of the planets in the sky as they relate to the natal chart, which is fixed in place like a snapshot of the heavens at the moment of birth.) Transits of the outer planets—Saturn, Uranus, Neptune, and Pluto—have the most influence because they move slowly through the signs of the zodiac. This long-term effect represents major changes in life development—a carrying out of the entelechy, or inner plan of one's life, of which crises, including illness, are a part. The passage of one or more of these planets over a major point in the natal chart—principally the Sun, Moon, or one of the angles—constitutes a *transforming crisis* during which period one is presented with the opportunity—often the *necessity*—to make life-changing decisions, often with profound effects.

Swiss astrologer Alexander Ruperti, in *Cycles of Becoming*, describes the crisis as symbolized by astrological concepts as follows:

> Cycles are measurements of change. In order for any purpose to be realized, change must take place, and change necessarily involves crises. Many have difficulty with the word *crisis*, confusing it with "catastrophe." [However]...it derives from the Greek word *krino*, "to decide," and means simply *a time for decision*. A crisis is a turning point—that which precedes CHANGE.

Healing Mind, Body, Spirit

If crises and the attendant need for change are not fully met, the person will remain caught in what Joseph Campbell has called "the nursery triangle" of dependence on the established family and social patterns. Locked in this pattern and unable to realize the SELF, evolution further of the implicate order is impossible.

This is not to say that failure is doom. There is always another chance; if one crisis is not met adequately, another will present the problem in a different guise until the sufferer finally gets the message. An outer planet transit is therefore a momentous time, revealing a person's individual pattern. Jung called these inner dynamics, represented by the planets, *archetypes*; we can also think of them as *planetary vibrations* to which we resonate at many different levels of our SELF. When we work with our implicate plane during outer-planet transits, we are tuning into the healthy and unimpaired patterns that underlie our being, express our individuality, promote healing, and engender spiritual growth by connecting us to the cosmic organism.

Medical astrology—that is to say the charting of medical conditions and/or diagnosis—is a specialty I do not practice. However, anyone who is interested in his or her overall health, or challenged by an illness, would do well to investigate his or her chart. By checking transits, which may have a long duration of influence, one may be able to see cosmic indications that correlate with the condition being observed.

The knowledge that a particular transit is finite can be of great help. When a difficult experience can be pinpointed, in relation to one or more transits of the outer planets, information about the duration and nature of the crisis is gained. These periods cover anywhere from one to several years after the onset of the problem. Equally, one can use knowledge of transits to identify time periods of elevated stress, lowered vitality, or susceptibility to infection.

~ Transits of Saturn

Saturn is known as the Lord of Karma—of restrictions, limitations, lessons to be learned. These transits are not easy ones and can bring on illness characterized by constriction, debilitation, or hardening. Transits of Saturn to the planets of the natal chart represent areas of your life that are being challenged and behavior patterns that require examination, and, quite possibly, change. Any illness occurring during a Saturn transit is likely to be necessary in the sense that it points out that you can no longer ignore what needs to be done. Most people experience Saturn's energies as if an external force beyond their control overtakes them; however, this is not the case. The unconscious mind, in reaction to the conscious mind refusing to take the required action, programs the event that precipitates the reevaluation that is the prerequisite to change. A Saturn transit puts you in touch with your *real* needs. Often people who experience loss or illness under a Saturn transit "see the light," and are empowered to make alterations to their viewpoints and live more in accordance with who they really are.

Many of the major crises of adulthood are represented by the energy of Saturn—tough times when one has to make a decision to forgo one path in favor of another. Saturn is *reality*—it is the need for duty and discipline, and who does not learn these twin lessons is never fully adult. Reality is *structure*, and structure is Saturn's province. Reality means limitations—this, but not that; one thing, but not the other. To master Saturn is to master necessity.

Transits of Saturn urge one on toward maturity. They tend to focus one's concern on areas of life that need work, and the crises they bring serve to force the issues that need attention, especially if they have been ignored or neglected. Saturn is also known as the Great Teacher, and often guides will appear under a Saturn transit. These can come in many guises, human and otherwise. Sometimes illnesses serve as teachers and guides, for when we are ill and dealing with healing we discover insights about ourselves. Many find inner strengths they didn't know they possessed. Others, like LeShan's cancer patients, are liberated through a "turning point," which lets them live more fully, in greater harmony with themselves and their families, friends, and communities. The lessons of Saturn are difficult—but they are necessary and worthwhile.

Saturn rules the bones and teeth, and his transits often signal problems in these areas. An astrologer friend was approaching a Saturn transit to her Sun in Aries (Aries rules the head), and so decided it was time for a dental checkup. Her dentist discovered an incipient problem that was corrected easily, but had she not been aware of the possibility of tooth trouble, she would have postponed visiting the dentist and had a major condition later on.

As Saturn holds back energy, its transits can indicate blocks of various kinds as well as difficulty with joints or broken bones. Another friend fell and broke her hip while Saturn was affecting her chart. She had been overworking for a long time, endangering her health, but could not be persuaded to take time off to rest. Saturn presented her with several weeks in bed, and she got her much-needed rest.

~ Transits of Uranus

Saturn's structure can become rigidity; discipline can narrow to stricture; necessity can become stultifying; order, a prison; duty, total lack of spontaneity. Uranus is an antidote to the calcifications of Saturnine reality. It gleefully knocks down those rigid structures, sending everything tumbling about.

The energy of Uranus is *unexpected*, sudden, and often disruptive. Uranus represents the desire to break free of limitations—its energy works to keep things flexible by preventing too

The Transforming Crisis

much unbending order. It is the random element of creativity. Uranian forces strive to break a person out of old, outworn patterns that have become rigid and too limiting. Order is necessary, but the "old order" must always give way to a new one. The power of Uranus comes in to transform and restructure lives in ways that are more fulfilling, opening the person up to new, sometimes alien, realities. Uranian energy seems to strike particularly when a person has become stuck in the status quo, unsatisfied and discontent, but not knowing how to make the needed changes, firing an urgent need to break free of the restrictions that have been limiting further development.

The individual who makes friends with Uranus in the chart and heeds the transits of this electrifying planet is one who will continue growing throughout life. The person who resists change, who is utterly dependent upon the regularity and predictability of the status quo, will have much difficulty encountering a transit of Uranus. But change must come, or we become calcified in the old, outworn pattern. Uranus will not allow attachment to the status quo, as is demonstrated by what happened to one of my clients. This man knew he needed to make major changes but was resisting taking action. He was under strong influence from a transit of Uranus, but although he acknowledged the urgency intellectually, his inflexible nature made change difficult for him to handle. Seeing the possibility of a disruptive occurrence, I begged him to get on with what he knew he needed to do. Still he resisted.

At that time, he was locked in a contest of wills with his wife, who was also his business partner. She too knew that change was needed but disagreed with him about the nature and direction of the change. At last, almost as a diversionary tactic, he decided to move his offices to another building, a matter of contention between them. He realized he was being unnecessarily stubborn and intractable, not facing the real issues, but, disregarding his wife's opposition, he went ahead with his plan.

On moving day, as he was carrying the first box of supplies down the stairs of his old office to his car, *he fell and broke both arms*. Uranus had ruthlessly shattered his Saturnine structure in a most dramatic way. Now, without his wife's help, he could not move his office, and in the wake of the accident he had no choice but to confront the real issues and resolve them.

During the enforced period of recuperative inactivity, in the absence of conjured-up distractions, he sorted out his priorities. His wife, forced to attend to his needs, was able to make compromises she previously had been unwilling to consider. One can say that this accident could have been prevented, but, given the man's innate psychological constitution (his implicate order), one could also make the case that there was no other way to pry open his resistance.

Recognizing this power of Uranus to force change in a drastic way allows one to be prepared to take advantage of this energy's structure-annihilating opportunities. If we knowingly dismantle our old structures willingly, to make room for the change that must come, we will not suffer the more serious effects of the transit. It is only when we resist, as my client did, that drastic action is taken. With a Uranus disruption, we have the opportunity to search through the rubble for what is worth keeping and chuck out the garbage from our psychic storeroom.

A case in point is the sudden onset of the symptoms of cancer that hospitalized me for surgery: I had visited the doctor in the afternoon; alarmed because he knew my history, he sent me home to pack and get to the hospital that night; the next morning at dawn I was on the operating table. Uranus was transiting my mid-heaven point (the top of the vertical axis, or an angle). This point is the cusp of the tenth house, and the tenth house signifies the mother.

The sheer dramatic jolt of this totally unexpected surgery, which resulted in my discovery that my mother had *not* died of reproductive-organ cancer, changed my previous concept of reality dramatically. It served to break up old inner structures, calcified in childhood, that were causing me multiple emotional and physical problems. Once a person has faced the need for a new view of reality, new structures can be built that are consonant with the person's true SELF.

Uranus, for all his ability to intrude harshly upon our dearly beloved status quo, is a friend. His powers can re-create aliveness and re-establish touch with the core of our being that has been concretized by Saturn's structure. It's a fact that people feel exhilarated when facing an emergency. For some reason, dealing with disaster brings out the best and the most creative in human beings. A Uranian transit may not be easy, but it is a good tonic for hardening of the attitudes.

A spasmodic energy, Uranus can distort bodily rhythms, especially in women. Anyone under a Uranus transit should be careful to get proper rest and keep calm. Nervousness and mental tension are related to Uranus, and these can cause stress-related illnesses such as headaches, digestion problems, or spastic episodes. Accidents are a possibility and, as in the case given, can result from the suppression of this energy. Physical tension, general strain from increased stress, cardiovascular difficulties, psychosomatic illness, and nervous disorders all occur under transits of Uranus. Relaxation exercises, physical exercise, and recognition of the need to make necessary changes in one's life are the antidotes. Often these transits affect people who are mostly cerebral and force them to get more in touch with their bodies. A Uranus transit is a good time to learn meditation techniques that facilitate this.

~ Transits of Neptune

Neptune is perhaps the most difficult planetary energy to understand. It is associated with all that is diffuse, illusory,

Healing Mind, Body, Spirit

vague, otherworldly, imaginative, psychic. Transits of Neptune can be especially difficult because of the vagueness of the effects. Under a Neptune transit, symptoms can be hard to diagnose or a condition can develop that resists treatment because the symptoms are unspecific.

Another effect of Neptune can be a desire to abdicate responsibility for one's self, to have others take care of you. Vague indefinite symptoms can send people from doctor to doctor, looking for someone to "understand" and provide care. The opposite of this is someone who, under a Neptune transit, utterly disregards his or her own needs and takes care of others to the extent of self-damage. There is a breakdown of the ego-structure under a Neptune transit, and it can be accompanied by feelings of defeat, confusion, and apathy. Mental conditions, such as depression, are a possibility under Neptune, as are addictive behaviors.

Depending upon the person's level of consciousness, a Neptune transit can also bring into play feelings of exhilaration and an opening up to a sense of being at one with all life, with the Universe. There can be a feeling of being "out of this world," because Neptune is outside time and space, symbolizing the "other," a dimensionless or multidimensioned universe.

Illness that occurs during a Neptune transit usually has the effect of being ego-annihilating. This is because the ego dissolves in Neptune's vapors. Under his influence, one comes to realize that the ego is not ultimately real. This realization, if encountered in the right spirit, liberates by promoting detachment from over-identification with the physical self and its concerns. With Neptune, we are in touch with the *ideal real*, which transcends physical reality and lets us understand that "I am not my body." We come to know that the essential SELF is boundless and limitless.

As the planet of mystics, seers, visionaries, and the transcendent realm, Neptune represents the level where individuality

The Transforming Crisis

is merged into universality: the Infinite. Neptune's energies have little to do with the physical universe. Many people have had visionary, ecstatic, miracle-cure, and near-death experiences under Neptune's influence.

Persons who are heavily dependent upon a prescribed structure to contain their lives will be most disturbed by a Neptune transit, for it can fog over everything and make the most solid-seeming of structures turn to ungraspable mist. Being ungrounded is extremely difficult for these types, who may think they are becoming mentally ill. Those with a somewhat weak ego may fare best under a Neptune transit, for they have less to hold on to. They are more sensitive to the transformative energies coming through them, to which others deny a place in their rigid reality systems.

Neptune is involved with the immune system as well as with the emotional body, and his effects can cause lowered vitality. Often someone with a Neptune transit just wants to sleep and dream, which is a good idea because it puts the person in touch with his or her implicate order.

Under Neptune transits, people tend to lose touch with ordinary reality and get in touch with extraordinary realities. I have had considerable personal experience with this energy and can attest to its effects. The period of my most intense psychic development took place under a major Neptune transit of several years' duration during which time I was beset by a multitude of ephemeral symptoms and an overwhelming need for sleep.

Neptune is a great teacher and bringer of higher consciousness and, though this can manifest merely as escapism (often through drugs and alcohol), his transits give us an opportunity to develop insight into our real needs. It is a time when we are naturally inclined to turn to more holistic methods of healing. This often evolves from the need to spend

Healing Mind, Body, Spirit

time alone to sort through the confusion experienced under a Neptune transit. With Neptune, we have the impetus to get to the root of what is amiss in our lives, both psychically and physically, and to seek out a positive therapy that suits our unique needs. Under Neptune, conditions can vanish as mysteriously as they presented, with no apparent cause either for the onset or the resolution.

Transits of Pluto

Pluto is *the* planet of transformation. More than any other influence—and his transits last the longest—he indicates the process of transformation that is healing. Ruler of Scorpio, the sign of the physician, Pluto can either bring on a health crisis or resolve a long-standing condition. Pluto is god of the underworld; under his influence hidden things are flushed out into the open to be dealt with.

One of the most dramatic instances of this was a client, a young gay man, who said he came to consult me "to find out about my Moon." Analyzing his chart prior to our meeting, I saw he was under a major Pluto transit. I wondered what had really motivated him to seek counsel. When he arrived and was seated, I said I was surprised that his interest in astrology seemed so casual as the Pluto transit indicated a major life crisis. At this, he burst into tears and emotionally confessed that he had just been given a diagnosis of AIDS. He was in a state of terror because his ultra-religious, uptight family did not know he was gay, and he feared being rejected by them in his desperate hour. After our session, he realized that he needed to "fess up" to his reality, to be true to his SELF, whatever the price. This was a hard lesson, but it served the purpose of reconciling him to his family and bringing a full measure of peace to him about who he really was.

The Transforming Crisis

Pluto represents the regenerative process, the total makeover we give ourselves after "hitting bottom" in some area of our lives. It marks the rebirth we experience when we finally say "nevermore" to past patterns of self-destructive behavior and negative thinking. Unlike the suddenness of Uranus, Pluto is subtle—its evolutionary power works slowly and at great depth, permeating the psyche, replacing old aspects of the personality with new ones in a process of fundamental transformation. With Pluto, refusal to deal with bodily or emotional realities can manifest as serious illnesses, while the need to transform—both emotionally and physically—provides the opportunity to make far-reaching changes, to replace the old with the new.

Pluto rules elimination—if you do not eliminate your bodily wastes, your own toxicity poisons you. It is the same with psychic waste. It must be eliminated to make room for the new growth. A crab sheds its shell in order to grow larger; the serpent, one of the animal symbols of Scorpio, which Pluto rules, sheds its skin—a characteristic that has identified it with the process of death and rebirth. The Moon, also, symbolizes this process, "dying" each month to be "reborn" as the shining silver crescent. These are Plutonian processes. They are inherent in the growth patterns of the human psyche. There will always come times when the psyche, and the body, must undergo crises involving breakdown and regeneration.

Pluto symbolizes the end of the process begun with Saturn. First, reality is structured; then Uranus comes along and knocks down the outdated structure; Neptune dissolves resistance and exposes us to the ultimately real dimension. Finally, Pluto brings on the radical transformation of consciousness that results in our being "reborn" into the spirit. Pluto can be compared to the Hindu god Shiva, who dances the world into being and then destroys it. Both creator and destroyer, Shiva is the god of rebirth and regeneration, the archetype of death and resurrection. Pluto works to break down the old and outworn patterns into their basic components, and then reassembles them into new and revivified being. When we encounter Pluto transits, we confront aspects of ourselves that are difficult to deal with because we have overlaid them with "the ordinariness of life," buried them under the structure of every day.

Unfortunately, people with a Pluto transit tend to become overwhelmed by the pain of the situation and resort to tranquilizing drugs, which only slows the breakdown-and-decay process and prolongs the agony. While I do not recommend that anyone forgo getting help for any condition, especially a mental one, I do think it is always wise to think carefully before submitting to drug therapy, which can mask the needs of the SELF and delay or even prevent the rebuilding process.

Pluto refers to a metaphorical death, something that ceases to be. Sometimes what must be allowed to die are things we hold on to from the past—hopes, dreams, memories, cherished ambitions—especially those involving other people. We can be held back from fully living our lives by these anchors to the past.

For example, in the wake of a Plutonian breakdown, I suffered an intense depression and, like many others, I sought psychiatric help. The "help" I was given was prescription antidepressant drugs, which I instinctively knew to avoid. Nevertheless, since I had never taken any drugs of this type, I followed the prescribed routine, getting no relief at all. In fact, I got worse and began having panic attacks. Alarmed, I decided it would be better to deal with the situation on my own and stopped taking the drugs.

Plunging into my own labyrinthine depths unaided, I stopped trying to find an antidote for my pain and allowed myself to experience it. In time, I found the root of my pain and expunged it. It was an old, old hanging-on to a part of my life that had died many years ago. I excavated the decaying remains of the past and put them to rest. The drugs were a hindrance, not a help.

Sometimes the state of total surrender activates the energy needed to effect healing. The hour before the dawn is always the darkest. And, with Pluto, we are already regenerating, even in the midst of our suffering, though we can't see clearly what the transition is bringing.

A concert pianist injured his hand and was no longer able to play. For several years, he wallowed in self-pity, doing nothing except lamenting lost glory. Finally, under a Pluto transit, he suffered a suicidal depression that forced him to examine other possibilities. He began to compose and realized that he had actually been bored with performing the same famous concerti over and over, season after season. He began to study the musical literature for the left hand and eventually returned to the concert hall. At the premiere of his own left-hand concerto, which he performed and which was hailed by the critics, he said to an interviewer, "I feel reborn."

Often, a Pluto transit will bring events or conditions that act as a mirror of something that did not get handled in the past, at the appropriate time. This can be a reference to a recurrent or chronic ailment. It is only by confronting that past and resolving it that coping with the present is possible. A Pluto crisis is an opportunity to *transform old unwanted problems* into new life energy. Health comes from the willingness and commitment to undergo this process.

Of course, it is difficult to see that our pain has a purpose, especially when we are immersed in the problem. It is much easier to run for the tranquilizers and antidepressant drugs—and our quick-fix society encourages us to do so. In our myopic demand for instant relief, we cannot see far enough to realize that the reason for the pain is the need for the old to work its way out of the system. An experience of mine will illustrate the point.

At nineteen, I had my wisdom teeth removed. Ten years later, I suffered excruciating pain that I identified as a toothache. An emergency dental visit and an X-ray showed nothing in the molar. The dentist could not say what was causing the pain, which grew worse. He prescribed codeine, but it did not help. Over the New Year's holiday, I lay in bed and suffered intensely. I had never experienced such pain. As one does with a sore tooth, I kept exploring the area with my tongue, which caught on a sharp point in the gum. After another two days, a small, needle-sharp sliver worked its way through the gum and the pain vanished. It was a bit of bone not removed properly during the wisdom-tooth surgery, and it had spent ten years working itself out to be discarded. The pain was its journey out of my body. What I suffered coping with chronic fatigue syndrome and the severe depression that accompanied it was like that bone sliver—the pain was intense but in the end something deeply embedded in my system that was causing damage was brought to the surface and eliminated.

Pluto transits may be experienced on many levels, depending on one's level of consciousness. The energy is hardest to handle for those bound up in the meat-and-potatoes structures of Saturn. A force beyond the ego, Pluto operates with extreme power—often manifesting as power struggles. It can cause you to feel totally out of control. Uranus disrupts ordinary reality; Neptune confuses it; but Pluto breaks it down completely. Ruling death and decay as well as regeneration, Pluto transits can bring a sense that everything is disintegrating around you.

If those undergoing Pluto transits can accept the need for building a new reality, rather than desperately trying to maintain the old structure, the process is less upsetting. Attempting to hold on to the old strains reserves and can bring on illness, especially of a mental nature. The time comes when the old structures no longer work. They cannot be repaired or patched up any longer. The only choice is to destroy them and rebuild. The best advice I can give to those having a Pluto transit is to let go of whatever must be let go in order to hasten the birth of the new.

People who have integrated the energies of Pluto often assist others who are going through such transformations. This positive aspect relates Pluto to healers and therapists, both psychological and physical, and to those who teach techniques of self-transformation. I write this book while Pluto is transiting my Sun. Spiritual leaders who espouse rebirth, either literal or metaphorical, are also expressing Pluto's message of rebirth into Spirit.

While transits are in effect, the information about what is going on may reach us merely as a vague sensation, either mental or emotional. It can be a tension or a sense that something is about to happen. Consciousness may register no more than an ephemeral state of being, like feeling that one has forgotten something important. Issues working themselves out from the implicate to the explicate order may bypass consciousness altogether and be expressed as an organic disturbance, a changed hormonal output, a headache, or a cold. Reaching into our intuitive realm can help to put us in touch with what we need to know.

So much of our everyday life is such a blur of routine that we miss what is going on at the deeper levels of our SELF. To combat this tendency, use the monitoring technique, which is a way of consciously focusing on the day's input, either as it is happening or during brief periods of reflection.

The Monitoring Technique

Begin by *consciously* storing in memory your thoughts, feelings, and reactions to the events of the day, especially those preceding or during an illness. For example, if you feel a cold coming on, review the events leading up to the sensation of a congested head or a sore throat.

If you have trouble remembering, train yourself to take brief notes during the day at or following significant events, especially negative ones. Note the particulars of the situation along with your reactions. A few words will do—you will develop a kind of shorthand in time. The purpose is to give your memory a jog later and enable you to recall the entire event with its "feeling tone."

When thoughts and feelings arise from the inner self, do not ignore them or push them away; record them either in writing or memory, so that they do not vanish in the well of forgetfulness. During the day, whenever you have a spot of unoccupied time—waiting for a bus, sitting on a train, standing in line—review what you have noted to fix it firmly for later evaluation.

At the end of the day, set aside a few minutes to examine the entire day's input for insights about your inner workings, clues to your implicate order. The more you are aware of these constantly ongoing processes, the better equipped you are to heal yourself at the onset of any disturbance in your SELF, either in body or in psyche.

The Transforming Crisis

While each of us is in the process of working out our inherent life pattern, it is essential to realize that "self-created" illness is not the result of any *conscious* doing. These malign incursions into the physical realm from the deep, unconscious imprint of negative experience, by no means the fault of the sufferer. To blame ourselves, asking what we did wrong, is to miss the point entirely—and is counterproductive to the genuine healing engendered by the process of transformation. In fact, by placing blame, and adding shame into the bargain, the poisonous fumes of guilt are released into the system, further toxifying it and delaying or even preventing the helpful insights from doing their healing work.

The transforming crisis signals that healing has *already begun*. Like a boil appearing on the skin, it represents toxins coming to the surface, ready to be released from the system so that healing can be completed. A fever always peaks just before it breaks, and the healing crisis can bring on an intensification prior to being resolved.

It's important to keep this in mind as you use the healing techniques. Reexperiencing past wounds in order to put them into the proper perspective can be painful, even more painful at times than the presenting illness, but while the pain is temporary, the healing is permanent. It may be necessary to seek and receive treatment, but it makes no sense to attempt to mask reality by the use of substances that may only serve to either shut down the healing process or delay it. The transforming crisis is there for a purpose: it puts us on notice that change is mandatory. Most of us won't make those changes unless we are forced to—the heart patient doesn't alter his or her lifestyle until an attack occurs; the smoker doesn't quit until a lesion is found on the lung; the chronic worrier resists relaxation until an ulcer is diagnosed; and so forth.

Fortunately, the healing crisis often happens well in advance of serious damage or illness and, if heeded and worked with, can serve to prevent or ameliorate severe physical breakdown. By dealing with the underlying emotional content at the time we become aware of the need, instead of thrusting it away from our awareness, we are often able to circumvent more serious consequences. By thoughtful reaction and the avoidance of any attempt to bypass the process, we open the way to our healing. Here are some affirmations you can use with any transit.

I face the prospect of change with acceptance.
I know that as one door closes, another opens.
I let go of the past and trust in a better future.
The future does not frighten me. I face it fearlessly.
I trust in my own Spiritually Evolving Life Force.
I let go all old, outworn patterns and behaviors.
I always expect a miracle.

In *Death and Reincarnation: Eternity's Voyage*, the buddhist sage Sri Chinmoy sums up the essence of outer-planet transits and the crises they symbolize beautifully. He says,

> At every moment we are dying and renewing ourselves. Each moment we see that a new consciousness, a new thought, a new hope, a new light is dawning in us. When something new dawns, at that time, we see that the old has been transformed into something higher, deeper, and more profound.

chapter ten
The Healing Moon

The moon, as the luminous aspect of the night, belongs to [the Goddess]; it is her fruit, her sublimation of light, an expression of her essential spirit. [It] appears as a birth—and indeed as rebirth. Such processes are the primordial mysteries of the Feminine...from which all life arises and unfolds, assuming, in its highest transformation, the form of the spirit.

— Erich Neumann
The Great Mother

Physicist David Bohm speaks of a "link or bridge between realms." Astrologically the Moon represents the *Soul*, which is the link between Spirit (Sun) and Matter (Earth). The Moon is feminine: it represents what we *feel* and how we *respond*. Therefore, it is emblematic of all that is *receptive* in human nature: the subconscious; the emotions; the behavioral instincts; the automatic functions of the body, such as the autonomic nervous system, digestion, breathing, and the like.

What Dr. Larry Dossey calls "an inner source of healing and strength that operates behind the scenes," I term the *lunar self*. As the channel for the flow of the universal, or divine, source, the Moon has great healing power.

In our society, we give far more weight to the Sun, or masculine-rational, functions of ourselves than we do to the Moon, or creative-nonrational, functions. What is valued most are the traditional *masculine* traits of action and rational, linear thinking. Although these feminine lunar traits are vital to our well-being—such crucial issues as dependency and nurturing, our sense of security and safety, and the ability to relate emotionally are the Moon's domain—they are not highly valued by our dominantly solar culture. It's the hustling salesman, the profit-driven executive, the hard-nosed lawyer, the tough politician, the professional athlete who gets the attention, the money, and the applause. And the heart attacks. And a host of other ills. When we become too involved with our Sun energy, we tend to neglect or deny our Moon energy and throw ourselves out of balance, individually and collectively.

However, anyone can be a lunar type. Donna Cunningham, a social worker who is also a brilliant astrologer, notes in her book *Being a Lunar Type in a Solar World* that she has observed many people who are disconnected from their lunar selves because of pressures to conform to the solar world around them. They are taught to consider themselves out of step with the norm.

Despite voluminous evidence that children who are not given sufficient nurturing grow into adults with a wide range of personal and social problems, the function of nurturing is low on society's totem pole of values. However, Moon needs are vital to health and well-being, and when these go unmet, you become unhappy at the deepest core of your being—a sure precursor to illness, sometimes of the sort called "psychosomatic." These Moon needs stretch back to the time when you were in the cradle and dependent on others for your survival needs: nourishment, warmth and cleanliness, a sense of safety and well-being, and, most important, love and affection.

The Moon is best understood in terms of basic emotional needs, habit patterns, bodily rhythms, and what makes us feel comfortable. Its role is important both in analyzing where illness may arise and how healing may be effected.

The Moon in your chart is the area of your life where old conditioning from childhood resides. It shows patterns that are as old as you are, from the days when you were rocked and held and given love and affection—or deprived of these vital necessities. It is a knee-jerk place within you that ticks off old patterns—your personal implicate order that manifests both in your body and in your psyche. It symbolizes what is most basic to you, thus pointing the way to healing. The Moon shows how you take care of yourself and others and, by extension, how you want to be taken care of when you are in need of healing.

Interestingly, the Moon does not revolve around the Earth alone—Earth and her Moon revolve *around each other*. This is a symbolic fact of great significance because it indicates a mutuality and interdependence that is mirrored in our lives in the implicate/explicate order.

Long before you were able to think or express yourself in words, you learned what to *feel* and how to *respond*. Much of how we understand ourselves to be was imprinted at a very early age. Based on the feeling-tone attached to both what we found pleasurable and threatening, our self-understanding became automatic behavior. We have been "conditioned" so repeatedly that by now we have ingrained *reactions*, of which we are almost totally unaware. As an illustration, think of something that revolts you or attracts you. Where did that response come from? Were you repeatedly told that something was bad for you or good for you? Much of what is conditioned behavior has its roots in survival value. Whether you have duplicated your parents' or other caregivers' attitudes or whether you have had to improvise your own, we all have a set of defense mechanisms in play to some extent, and these are based on our lunar selves.

Neglect of the lunar self reaps a harvest of health-threatening conditions, most of which are seeded in the emotional body. We have already said that emotional distress of whatever kind, be it trauma or repression, guilt or shame, takes a serious toll on physical health. You, as an individual, however, can call upon the healing power of the Moon by becoming acquainted with your lunar self.

Knowledge of your Moon and how it operates will give you insight into your characteristic emotional responses and the feelings you are likely to repress, which, driven underground, can fester into both emotional and physical sickness. Home, family, mother, security, emotions, and food are all in the Moon's arena. By paying attention to and honoring our lunar selves and their needs, we can make quicker, more positive adjustments to ill health or trauma. You can find your Moon Sign in Appendix III.

The Moon through the Signs

Aries

You need to excel, always wanting to be first. Active and vital, you rush headlong into activities and love to take chances. Easily bored, you need frequent changes in routine and are happiest when busy. *Independence* is your key word. Frustration and being restricted are likely trouble spots. Aries rules the head, brain, and eyes, and you are susceptible to high fevers, headaches, and nervousness. You need to learn relaxation and meditation in order to "turn off" the thinking motor.

Taurus

You are serene. Your emotions function with a high degree of stability. Physical comfort is what you need the most. Security-conscious, you do not readily tolerate change and hang on fiercely—both to the past and possessions. *Mine* is your key word. Disrupted routines and being rushed are likely trouble spots. Taurus rules the neck, throat, and ears and has an affinity with the lymphatic system of the body and the thyroid gland. Metabolic processes may be slow, resulting in weight gain, and you are especially prone to sore throats when upset or blocked. In general, you seek practical solutions.

Gemini

You are bright, quick, witty, and changeable, flipping from mood to mood with astonishing rapidity. You hate boredom and need mental stimulation, especially conversation. Curious, you thrive on diversity and distraction. *Change* is your key word. Being cooped up, limited, or cut off from communication with others are likely trouble spots. Gemini rules the hands, arms, and much of the nervous system so nervous exhaustion can be a problem, especially when you are in a state of unsatisfied restlessness. Often the cure for what ails you is more diversion, but you also need to learn how to be quiet and rest.

Cancer

You are emotionally supersensitive and need nurturing and support all your life. Family is all-important, and separation from them is painful. Independence comes late. Food is a focus—it represents comfort and security. *Emotional* is your key word. Insecurity and feeling unloved are trouble spots. Cancer rules the chest and breasts and sensitivity to touch. Your body is delicate, even when full-blown, and you have a propensity toward catching colds and minor ailments, which gives you the opportunity to cuddle up with familiar things around you, be cozy, and pamper yourself—a sure cure.

Leo

You are warm and affectionate, so receiving plenty of affection makes you feel wanted and important. You crave attention, and histrionics is a favored method of achieving this end. A born ham, you need positive feedback. *Attention* is your key word. Lack of fun, praise, and acknowledgment are likely trouble spots. Leo rules the heart and possesses remarkable vitality and recuperative powers, but neglect and absence of love can cause illness. Overdoing can bring on physical collapse or burnout. What is needed to avoid this is an even pace to allow you to function in accord with your nature.

Virgo

You are fundamentally neat, even fussy. Cleanliness and orderliness are vital. Generally self-sufficient, when ill you crave to be nursed tenderly. Otherwise, you are self-contained, careful and meticulous, and naturally helpful, liking to achieve practical results. *Useful* is your key word. Disorder, dirt, and having your efforts ignored or not appreciated are likely trouble spots. Virgo rules the intestines and digestive system, and illness often attacks these functions. There are two types: those who fuss endlessly over health and those who practice self-neglect. Both need to get in touch with their sensuous nature and learn to let go of control.

Libra

You appreciate peace and quiet in calm, beautiful surroundings, for you hate strife of any kind and will shrink from gross behavior and people. You seek balance and like refinement. *Harmony* is your key word. Repressed anger, the expression of which can be explosive, and refusal to face unpleasantness are likely trouble spots. Libra rules the kidneys, of which there are two. Without a companion, Libra is sad and sour. Being alone is intolerable and brings on various ailments, as do inharmonious relationships and dependency on the approval of others. You need to develop independence.

Scorpio

You have perhaps the hardest time of all the signs understanding yourself. Your emotions run so deep that often you cannot identify them. This gives you a reputation for secrecy. There is a tendency to allow personal affairs to develop along obsessive lines, with jealousy as a result. *Intense* is your key word. Holding grudges, brooding over hurts, and plotting revenge are likely trouble spots, as is possessiveness. Scorpio rules the reproductive and excretory functions. Being naturally retentive, constipation can be a problem, as can disorders of the generative organs.

Sagittarius

You are naturally upbeat and radiate an innate sense of optimism. As you expect everything to go well, you are a good patient when ill. Endlessly curious, you seek out answers to the universal philosophical questions. *Optimism* is your key word. Sports injuries from lack of proper precautions and travel mishaps in foreign lands are likely trouble spots. Sagittarius rules the thighs, which are powerful and can be large, a source of embarrassment to women especially, which can cause emotional pain and eating disorders. Traditional religious beliefs can limit ability to explore a larger spirituality and can block healing efforts accordingly.

Capricorn

You have a reserved and cautious nature, to the point of austerity and identify with material rather than spiritual values. Uncomfortable with feelings, you need much love to thaw that natural Capricorn coldness. *Responsibility* is your key word. The active seeking of money can bring on stress ailments. Inability to release stress and have fun are likely trouble spots. Capricorn rules the knees, the joint essential to climbing to the top of the mountain. To ward off illness, or cope with it when it comes, you need to develop faith in the Universal Plan and to cultivate a hopeful outlook. Pessimism brings with it the danger of giving up.

Aquarius

You are innately humanitarian, but in an impersonal way. You thrive on diversity and the unusual. Sometimes you are unnervingly detached and rational. You may be interested in UFOs or believe you have seen aliens. *Exploratory* is your key word. The need for freedom at all costs, emotional detachment, and lack of personal involvement due to fear are likely trouble spots. Aquarius rules the ankles and is the only human image in the zodiac. Almost exclusively mental, your gyrations of abstract thought can bring on exhaustion. Failure to manifest air-built castles in the real world can cause eruptions of impatience and despondency.

Pisces

You have a supersensitive nature that acts like a psychic sponge, soaking up the thoughts and feelings of others—often negative ones—with concomitant damage to the health. You are often vaguely ill, as you tend to float in and out of what we call "reality." *Sensitive* is your key word. Negative vibrations from others, difficulty relating to the "real" world, and drugs and alcohol are likely trouble spots. Pisces rules the feet, on which the Dance of Life depends. Vulnerable and easily hurt, prey to feelings of persecution and to neurotic tendencies, you need to learn to balance a profound inner life with the demands of the material world.

The recently developed science of neurolinguistic programming provides us with tools to "tune in" to our inner, implicate order through astrological components. Mary Orser and Richard Zarro, in their book *Changing Your Destiny*, have provided "attunements," expressed in the first person, which help to identify "your *I* with the *archetypal I*." According to Orser, the attunement "could be considered an *invocation*—invoking the archetype." She adds, "This would fit with the theory that the signs are morphic fields." According to the authors, these attunements are "extremely effective for connecting you with the [zodiacal] empowering energy, thus connecting you with the archetypal healing force. Their Moon Attunement follows.

> I am the Moon,
> Ruler of Blue shadows and moist silence in
> The Bowl of Heaven.
> I give form to creative force.
> I am Fertile Matter, which sustains and nourishes
> Seeds of solar life.
> I absorb the solar currents
> By being passive, feminine, and receptive.

~ *Healing Mind, Body, Spirit*

> I am the sentient substance
> Of instincts, memories, and desires
> Waiting to be impregnated
> By the light, heat, and power of the Sun's rays.
> I am the Great Mother.
> The ancient ones called me
> One thousand names of mystery.
> I am the Celestial Midwife
> Cherishing the Child of Divine Seed.
> Sister of the Sun, the caress of The Mother,
> I am the breast of Life,
> Lover of Lovers,
> The Wisdom of the waters,
> Of instinct and ancestral experience,
> Of nature and spirit, Fate and the motion of Time.
> I harbor the secret knowledge and power of Love,
> Of the subconscious, of immortality,
> Of inspiration and instinctive desire.
> Mother of Enchantresses and Magicians,
> I rule the function and form of matter,
> Rhythms of the body and fate of the soul,
> Where one has been and what one has yet to face.
> I am the Captor and Reflector.

What About Your Sun Sign?

Most of us are familiar with our Sun Signs (that's the answer you give when someone asks, "What's your sign?"). The Sun is important: it is at the heart of the chart.

To help my clients harmonize their lunar selves with their solar selves, I devised the following special meditation as part of my unique AstroVision™ series, which combines visualization techniques with astrological components.

How to Balance Sun/Moon Energies

Prepare for this exercise by first walking about and taking a good long stretch to loosen your muscles and ready yourself for an inner experience. Then, sit or recline in a comfortable position you can hold for ten or fifteen minutes. Loosen or remove any tight clothing and close your eyes. First, pay total attention to your breath, without making any changes; simply observe the breath coming in and going out for several minutes until you feel a sense of relaxation and unwinding.

Now, imagine yourself holding your Sun in one hand and your Moon in the other. You may want to do this with your hands outstretched, or in your lap, or whatever feels comfortable. Allow yourself to feel the weight of each of the "lights" you are holding, as if you were trying to discover the differences between them. Choose one and put the other down. Then, with both hands, turn your chosen light about in your hands as you would an object that is new to you. Feel the size, texture, weight of it. See if it has any other characteristics, such as smell or sound or color.

Spend a few minutes, or as long as you feel comfortable, with the first light, making friends with it as you might with a new puppy or kitten. Then put it down and take up the second light in your hands, repeating the procedure.

After familiarizing yourself with the two lights on an individual basis, feel intuitively how they relate to each other. See if you want to say anything to either or both. You may want to ask questions, find out the best way to use the energies, or see what each needs of you. You can ask the Sun or Moon if it feels fulfilled, or you can bring more of its energy

> into focus in your life. Ask how to do this. Do this procedure with both lights.
>
> Then, take them both up together, one in each hand, and see what happens. You may feel that they want to dialogue, or that they have something to give each other or work out together. Give them equal time.

The more often you do this exercise, the more you will be in touch with your inner Sun and Moon and their relationship to each other within you and in your life.

The Nurturing Moon

The Moon in astrology is a metaphor for all that is instinctive and reactive—from emotions to physical processes. It symbolizes our experience—positive or negative—of being mothered, of nurture, of support, of love. The Moon is your *needs*, what makes you *feel cared for*, and the environment in which you *feel most comfortable*. As you can see, it has a lot to do with your feelings.

When Moon needs are fulfilled in childhood, we gradually and naturally grow out of the state of dependence on others by learning to care for ourselves. However, children whose lunar needs are not met may as adults have great difficulty respecting and honoring those needs. They may not even be able to identify them. Children who are thus deprived can become immature adults, either forever "needy" or afflicted with self-deprivation. The Moon indicates how we react when upset; how we comfort and heal ourselves; what is most basic; and, often, what is most unconscious—sometimes uncontrollable, as in cases of eating disorders.

It is vitally important to get to know and respect and honor those feelings in order for the transformative process of healing to take place properly. It is also important to realize that astrology is not an exact science (though, neither is medicine or psychology). Your chart, however, can aid you to confirm *tendencies* and natural proclivities related to health and healing.

Food is a major issue for many in our culture, perhaps a majority. Eating disorders are rampant and even take the lives of young people, the overwhelming majority of whom are female. Those not starving themselves to be thin are often obese. What's wrong here?

For the obese, food, being lunar, serves as a substitute for emotional satisfaction, as a balm for anguished feelings, as a sedative for the sense of deprivation that literally gnaws away inside. This is also true for the bulimic, who painfully stuff themselves with all the food their stomachs can hold and then induce vomiting to expel the undigested food before it can either nourish them or be stored as fat. In both instances, food is used to satisfy the hunger pangs of the soul.

Overeating is often triggered by the response to a lunar crisis, which is characterized by the surfacing of repressed emotions, by a sense of insecurity and neediness, and by a strong desire to be taken care of. Almost anything relating to emotions and desires can bring this on—moving out of the parental home (college students often experience sudden weight gain or develop eating disorders); becoming a parent (women have an especially hard time losing weight gained in pregnancy); divorce or death of a spouse; the loss of a parent, especially the mother; moving to another town, city, or state; "empty nest" syndrome; getting married.

Less severe instances can also trip the overeating hammer. Losing a job and feeling worthless or mistreated; the breakup of a romance; an argument or fight with a spouse, parent (especially your mother), sibling, good friend, or your boss; family difficulties of all types. Feeling abandoned, unloved, unwanted, unappreciated, or neglected can all cause a lunar crisis.

Nearly everyone experiences lunar crises on a personal level. Any major change can bring one on, especially for women who nurture too much and whose lunar tanks "run on empty" as a result. A lunar crisis can make you vulnerable to emotional imbalance and to feelings of deprivation and insecurity; it can bring on minor ailments or major illness.

A lunar crisis is often the precursor to a particularly debilitating condition called *lunar burnout*. Donna Cunningham, in *Moon Signs*, has described the symptoms of lunar burnout, which results when you're called on to nurture others for long periods that leave you no room for nurturing yourself. Lunar burnout hits deep at the emotions, making you feel irrationally needy and resentful of others' demands. You feel helpless and desperately want someone to come along and take care of you. The person who is suffering from lunar burnout may cry spontaneously for no apparent reason.

A condition of feeling totally drained and exhausted, lunar burnout strikes mothers and caretakers, especially those who nurture for a living, such as teachers and health-care workers. People who suppress emotional needs—men in particular—can experience this burnout. Since the Moon is related to the menstrual cycle, severe PMS is a symptom of lunar burnout, as is weight gain. However, *anyone* can have a lunar burnout. As self-nurturing is frowned upon, and nurturing itself is low-rated in this society, we are all at risk.

At one time the Moon represented a deep source of connectedness with family ties and natural rhythms; now it is often a problem arena. Traditionally the fundamental guardians of elemental energy—hearthfires, the drawing of well water, primary source of food, maintenance of the dwelling place—women are connected to an inner, archetypal sense of the feminine principle, represented by the Moon, which gives them a more stable lunar core. By contrast, men, who tend to be disconnected from their lunar selves, are more susceptible to cracking during a lunar crisis. Less in touch with their own deep inner realms of feeling and instinct, they rely almost entirely on their solar selves and rational, linear thought. Very often they put their lunar selves into foster care—giving that part of themselves over to a woman to take care of while they devote themselves to their work and play.

Thus, they live in a state of denial about their dependency needs and tend to neglect signals from the body when something is wrong. There are serious consequences for this male abandonment of the lunar self. In all age groups, there is a far higher death rate for men than for women, and for fourteen of the fifteen leading causes of death, men have a higher death rate than women. On average, women outlive men by eight years, with this figure increasing.

Today, as more women move into the work force and take on roles previously reserved for men only, they, too, are becoming increasingly disconnected from their lunar selves. Once the keepers of the lunar flame, they now are forced to abandon the Moon-governed support systems while still performing the age-old lunar *functions* of housework and childcare, food procurement and preparation, and being the family's emotional bulwark.

The good news is that lunar burnout can be avoided. Since the Moon is the symbol of nurture, the solution is *self-nurture*, which can mend the lunar self. A note of caution: you can't get the nurturing you need from others—don't even try. This is strictly a do-it-yourself proposition.

My first prescription both for avoiding lunar burnout and for recovering from it is *self-love*—love of SELF. The fact is that we cannot really love another—though we may *serve* others well—if we cannot first love ourselves.

Being good to ourselves, recognizing that we deserve the same care and attention we give to our loved ones, and taking that understanding into *action* is the key to honoring the lunar self and the practice of self-nurturance. Not everyone wants to be nurtured in the same way, as a study of the Moon through the signs indicates. However, there are general guidelines that apply to all the Moon signs. Ask yourself these questions:

- Do I take time out each day for my own purposes?
- Do I derive my sense of worth largely through other people's approval or expression of gratitude?
- Do I try to get my own needs met by giving?
- Am I identified primarily with my caretaking abilities?

There are practical ways you can meet your needs, which involve physical, emotional, and spiritual modes. By giving yourself pleasurable and soul-satisfying experiences, you learn to feel good about yourself *by yourself*. Breaking the dependence on other people's responses is the key to self-nurturance. When we replace our self-negating habits with self-nurturing ones, we increase our overall health.

You may be asking, "What does treating ourselves well have to do with physical health?" The authors of *Healthy Pleasures*, Robert Ornstein, Ph.D., and David Sobel, M.D., answer this question with an unequivocal statement that "the healthiest people seem to be pleasure-loving, pleasure-seeking, pleasure-creating individuals." Citing scientific studies to support their views, these authors say that positive moods and emotions tend to enhance the immune system and have been associated with disease recovery. They recommend enhanced use of the five senses: *sight, sound, smell, taste, touch*.

While this is not the whole picture, these studies suggest that our nervous, immune, and cardiovascular systems respond to sensual experiences. Pleasing sights, mellifluous sounds, delightful fragrances, delicious tastes, and the pleasure of touch all serve to enhance our health and well-being.

Why do we feel guilty at pleasing ourselves? Why does taking time for purely personal pleasure seem like we are stealing it from someone else? Despite America's brief plunge into hedonism during the "sexual revolution" of the 1960s, our Puritan heritage hangs on tight, making us uptight about sensual pleasures. This is because we tend to equate sensual pleasure only with *sex*. We even speak of "sinful pleasures," as if pleasure itself were sinful, or of "guilty pleasures," implying that we should feel guilt when we enjoy ourselves.

Nurturing our senses leads to nurturing the inner self. The soul-satisfying pursuits of music, art, and literature not only promote health, they expand the range of our ability to appreciate life. With so many don'ts leaping at us from all sides, we are hard-pressed to admit a few dos into our lives. Ornstein and Sobel argue that even though it is politically correct to avoid many types of food and drink, these scorned "indulgences" are actually health-promoting when used in moderation, giving us a lift that resonates throughout the body-mind-spirit.

Our sight can be soothed by watching an aquarium full of tropical fish or by watching a movie. We do not have to go to a concert to hear beautiful sounds—we can listen to a bird's song and connect with nature. Our sense of smell can be pleasured in various ways—the scent of spiced apples was found to moderate the stress response, lower blood pressure, relax muscles, and slow heart rates. Wonderful tastes are widely available to those willing to experiment. Sweets are said to increase endorphins, the brain's natural pain-killing agent. And, if there's not a human handy, our sense of touch can be satisfied by stroking a furry pet.

Often, those who are sense-deprived are unaware of their lunar needs, denying themselves pleasures because they really believe they don't have time. Underlying this "no time" excuse is a basic feeling of being undeserving. "How can I take time for myself when _____?" You fill in the blank. Another factor in busy schedules is the fear that taking time for one's self is frivolous at best and unacceptably selfish at worst. This leads to guilt.

However, we bolster our general health and help ourselves to heal when we take care of ourselves on all levels—mentally, emotionally, physically, spiritually. It is time to stop denying this important fact and incorporate self-nurturance into our lives on a daily basis. Our health and well-being demand that we take care of our *whole* selves.

In a study of longtime survivors of AIDS by George F. Solomon, M.D., and Lydia Temoshok, Ph.D., an indicator to the healing potential of self-nurturance was uncovered. It was the willingness "to withdraw to nurture the self." Patients who did this had more suppressor cells, which help us to resist autoimmune diseases. Solomon and Temoshok's preliminary conclusion is that when we nurture our emotional, physical, and spiritual selves we also strengthen our immune system.

"Where will I find time to nurture myself?" is the most common response to the suggestion that a client begin to practice self-nurturance. My answer is always the same: We always find time for what we consider important. If I can convince you that self-nurturance is not only important but *absolutely vital* to your well-being, you will find the time for it. And, once you have begun to reap the benefits, you will find even more time. When you get sick, you "find the time" to be sick because you have no choice. So start making the healthy choice to find the time for yourself. Here are some tips to get you started. Not all of them will apply to everybody. Choose what suits your lunar nature. The key here is to find and activate what will give you pleasure, even in small amounts.

The Art of Self-Nurture

- Don't rush from bed to work in the morning. Take a few minutes to remember your dreams, meditate, think happy thoughts. Do something pleasurable for your senses before you start your day.
- Before leaving for your commute, do a mini-relaxation by taking time to pay attention to your breathing.
- If you drive to work, don't play the radio. Use a tape of nature sounds or just be with yourself.
- When stopped at a light or in traffic, look at the sky and trees and recall some affirmations.
- Before starting work, give yourself a few minutes of transition time. Plan to do monitoring.
- During breaks and at lunch, take the time for yourself. Take a slow walk alone or find a quiet place to meditate, such as a church or library.
- Take mini-relaxation breaks throughout the day, even if only for a few minutes.
- Put a flower on your desk or a plant in your office.
- When you ride the bus or drive your car at the end of the workday, take the time for monitoring.
- Congratulate yourself on what you have accomplished during your day. Plan tomorrow's work and then let work thoughts go.
- When you arrive home, change your clothing and wash your face before starting your evening. Refresh yourself with some sensual pleasure, such as a dash of cologne or a brief period of exercise.
- Don't rush through dinner, even if you have after-dinner obligations. Take the time to enjoy your food. Defer any unpleasant discussions for later.

Healing Mind, Body, Spirit

- Spend some time before bed pleasing yourself—soaking in a hot bath with scented water, reading, listening to music, writing in your journal, doing affirmations.
- Pamper yourself for at least half an hour every day.
- Make a list of things you would like to have in your life that would nurture you. Begin to bring them into being.
- Remind yourself that you *deserve* to have your needs met, and then meet them yourself.
- *Don't break promises to yourself.*

In addition to things you can do on a daily basis, here is a list of suggestions for long-term consideration.

- Treat yourself to a regular massage.
- Get a monthly pedicure.
- Try aromatherapy over a long weekend.
- Spend an entire day reading a book.
- Spend a weekend at a bed and breakfast in the country.
- Join a group or organization that appeals to you.
- Get a new hairstyle from a fashionable hairdresser.
- Take weekend nature walks, hikes, or camping trips.
- Don't go to the in-laws for the holidays this year.
- Buy something you really want but don't really need.
- Take a "psychological sick day" and play hooky.
- Call someone you miss long distance and talk as long as you want without worrying about the bill.
- Hire out some chore you really hate doing.
- Make a garden, indoors or out.
- Attend a weekend seminar.
- Take lessons in a subject you once loved but dropped, such as a foreign language or a musical instrument.
- Go dancing on a regular basis.
- Get a pet to love and care for.
- Spend an entire day indulging in goal-free activities.

- Take long walks on the beach at dawn or sunset.
- Learn to play.

Self-nurturance is an art because it requires us to do something we are totally unaccustomed to doing, and which seems unnatural because it means the *unlearning* of unwanted, negative behavior acquired in childhood, usually as a defense or survival mechanism. When you begin to fulfill your lunar needs, you will gain insights into your mother and her influence on your ability to nurture yourself.

Close examination usually shows that we nurture ourselves as we were nurtured—or not nurtured, as the case may be. If your mother took loving care of your physical and emotional needs—kept you clean and safe, fed and comfortable, and gave you lots of hugs and affection—the chances are that you have little problem nurturing yourself. If, on the other hand, she was impatient with your small needs, was absent for some reason, or griped and complained about all she had to do for you, you quite probably have neglected your lunar self all your life.

The basic human model is the mother, but for some people, it was a father, grandmother, or even a grandfather who played the mother role. Whomever your primary caregiver was, you will find an echo of that figure still active in you. Examine your attitude toward being sick and how you treat yourself when ill, and you'll most likely find the pattern of how your own mother treated you at such times. Her attitude toward *herself* will also be a factor. Did she take excellent care of you but neglect herself in the process? And do you today suffer from self-neglect? There is a connection.

Now we will look at the Moon through the signs in terms of how you can nurture and strengthen your lunar self. Each sign has both positive and negative characteristics. The less you are in touch with your lunar self, the more likely you are to be expressing its negative characteristics. You may immediately recognize yourself in the negative characteristics described. Don't worry. By becoming familiar with both sides of the lunar coin, you are in a better position to express the positive characteristics of your Moon sign. You can change by incorporating your own "self-nurturing highlight" into your life.

Learning to know and honor your lunar self is a *transformative experience*. It will change your life. And it will change the lives of those around you, usually for the better if they can but understand the importance of your mental, emotional, and physical health to *their* lives.

The Moon Through the Signs

Aries
Element: Fire

NEGATIVE— Aggressive, foolhardy, pushy, hotheaded, impatient, rushing, overbusy, impetuous.
POSITIVE— Action-initiating, pioneering, energetic, enthusiastic, decisive, courageous, active.

Your self-nurturing highlight is *physical exercise*, especially if you are a Fire Type. Sports that use a lot of energy, such as running and tennis, help you to work off excess emotional tension and replenish your overall vitality. Make a definite plan and set aside time each day for this purpose. As you have little patience with any personal need that interferes with what you want to do, you tend to ignore physical symptoms until they worsen or become serious. Your tendency to rush is another problem, as you don't take the time to eat properly. Take an active role in fighting off illness, as prevention will serve to keep the independence you value so highly, for when you are sick you become dependent on others.

Taurus
Element: Earth

NEGATIVE— Possessive, rigid, unyielding, stubborn, opinionated, materialistic, gluttonous.
POSITIVE— Stable, practical, productive, deliberate, affectionate, earthy, sensuous, artistic.

Your self-nurturing highlight is *green and growing things*, whether an outside garden or houseplants, especially if you are an Earth Type. Taurus is the quintessential earth-nature, and the Moon in Taurus is said to be in its *hipsoma*, "in honor." Astrologers say the Moon in Taurus is "exalted." Nurturing plants and soil will nurture *you*. Even if you only have a small window garden, make sure you have plants, especially flowering ones, in your environment. Go regularly to parks and nature spots, wilderness areas if you can reach them, to renew and refresh your lunar self. Food is important to you, but if weight is a problem you should establish a comfortable routine of light, healthy meals taken regularly to offset your tendency to indulge.

Gemini
Element: Air

NEGATIVE— Superficial, scattered, distracted, restless, trite, babbling, fickle, fidgety.
POSITIVE— Thinking, communicating, reasoning, curious, quick-witted, versatile, flexible, agile.

Your self-nurturing highlight is *talking with people you can trust*. This is a must for Gemini Moon who needs to "air" troubles and grievances at length. So what if your best friend or sister is on the opposite coast—splurge on the phone bill and you'll feel a lot better. You can cut corners elsewhere. Don't ever deprive yourself of this basic need to talk things out with a trusted friend. Action and thought are the twin pillars of

Healing Mind, Body, Spirit

Gemini, but it's easy to get stuck in the mental-only polarity. Offset this by sandwiching the necessary action in between discussing its pros and cons before and after.

Cancer
Element: Water

NEGATIVE— Oversensitive, insecure, clinging, illogical, acquisitive, self-indulgent, brooding, hoarding.

POSITIVE— Nurturing, feeling, caring, protecting, domestic, maternal, intuitive, devotional, sympathetic.

Your self-nurturing highlight is *proximity to water*. Cancer rules the Moon, and the Moon rules the ocean tides. Being near water, especially the sea, nourishes and refreshes you. The ceaseless undulation of the ocean feeds your soul and reconnects you to your element, especially if you are a Water Type. If you can't get to the ocean, find a stream to sit by or take frequent long soaks in the tub. Naturally nurturing, you may get so involved in the needs of others that you neglect your own important personal needs. If self-neglect is chronic, you tend to eat to excess sweet and starchy foods to soothe feelings of deprivation. Combat this by taking good care of yourself and preparing comforting, homemade meals. Also, frequent naps will serve to restore you to emotional balance.

Leo
Element: Fire

NEGATIVE— Self-centered, self-glorifying, willful, grandiose, overbearing, attention-getting.

POSITIVE— Loving, creative, loyal, courageous, leading, playful, childlike, warm, honorable, generous.

Your self-nurturing highlight is *getting out in the sun*, especially if you are a Fire Type. The natural warmth of Leo Moon can run cold during winter months or from too much time indoors. Getting out in the sun (the Sun rules Leo) will rejuvenate you. Make room in your budget for a vacation in the sun at least once each winter. You also need positive feedback from others, so ask for this, even though, since you don't like to show your needs or display "down" times, you may be reluctant to seek nurturance from others. Leo's pride gets in the way. Learn to stem your tendency toward lavish giving, especially if you are feeling blue or ill. Instead of picking up the check for the crowd, give to yourself: a massage, or a weekend at the beach.

Virgo
Element: Earth

NEGATIVE— Worrying, fault-finding, fussy, nit-picking, overcritical, nervous, introverted, self-effacing.
POSITIVE— Careful, orderly, discerning, discriminating, helpful, dutiful, meticulous, accurate, precise.

Your self-nurturing highlight is *letting up on perfectionism*. Into each life some dirt must fall, and though you do need an orderly and neat environment, you don't have to drive yourself crazy to get it. Accept that nobody is perfect, not even you, and learn to let others help so you aren't doing all the work yourself. Suspend critical judgment, learn to relax and just "hang out." The ceiling won't cave in if you take time off and let everything go to pot for a day or two. You must overcome your reluctance to self-nurture—it's not an indulgence; it's a necessity. You are usually so busy serving others that you drain yourself of health and vitality. Combat this by moving "self-care" from the bottom of your list of priorities to the top.

Healing Mind, Body, Spirit

Libra
Element: Air

NEGATIVE— Dependent on others' approval, inconsistent, indecisive, oppositional, judgmental, legalistic.
POSITIVE— Balancing, harmonious, diplomatic, appreciative, charming, graceful, considerate, socially aware.

Your self-nurturing highlight is *beauty in your environment*. A natural diplomat, you need peaceful surroundings, artfully decorated. Whether it is a vase of fresh flowers, a new slipcover, or a polished, beautifully arranged office, you respond to a calm and refined atmosphere. This is because Libra Moon is relational and needs a feeling of harmony in order to be in balance within. The food you eat should be visually appealing, and your home should be filled with music and beautiful things. You don't have to spend a lot of money—you can find wonderful treasures at thrift shops and flea markets. You need to do things in tandem, not alone, so find a buddy for your self-care: jogging, the health club, or artistic pursuits like concerts.

Scorpio
Element: Water

NEGATIVE— Relentless, secretive, coercive, vindictive, destructive, covetous, sarcastic, jealous.
POSITIVE— Transforming, regenerating, healing, intense, psychic, sexual, resourceful, determined.

Your self-nurturing highlight is *solitude*, especially around water, even if it's only in the bathtub. Time to be alone and regenerate yourself is of the utmost importance. Scorpio is the sign of the physician, and you have great recuperative powers, but your intensity and determination often do not allow you to use them on yourself. Because you are so strong, you tend to overdo, relying on your own amazing powers of self-rejuvenation. But if you let it go for too long, you could come down with a host of ailments, difficult to diagnose and treat. This is because when your transformative power is used negatively, you suffer the consequences. For Scorpio Moon, *forgiveness* is a must. Brooding on what has hurt you can make you sick.

Sagittarius
Element: Fire

NEGATIVE— Self-righteous, opinionated, exaggerating, blunt, hypocritical, judgmental, tactless, impractical.

POSITIVE— Understanding, far-seeing, expansive, optimistic, independent, athletic, travel-oriented, ethical.

Your self-nurturing highlight is *traveling*. Perhaps you cannot go off on a jaunt around the world, but recognize that you need travel to restore and refresh yourself. Make room in your budget for some trips, even if they are only short ones. Travel revitalizes Sagittarius Moon, who needs constant broadening of the horizons of thought and learning in order not to become stale and resentful. If you absolutely cannot travel, spend time with travel books, magazines, TV programs, and videos. And begin a travel savings account. Put away a few dollars every time you can for a future trip. Don't deny yourself this necessity. Sagittarius is the quintessential sign of optimism. For you, there is power in positive thinking. Use affirmations.

Capricorn
Element: Earth

NEGATIVE— Competitive, worrying, overstructured, stiff, restrictive, authoritarian, austere, severe.
POSITIVE— Achieving, organized, serious, practical, focused, self-controlled, professional, wise, efficient.

Your self-nurturing highlight is *learn to live in the present*. Security-conscious Capricorn Moon is always thinking of the future rainy day and fails to enjoy today's sunshine. Neglecting yourself in favor of working even harder to accumulate more protection against projected adversity, you do not relax and enjoy what you already have. *Relaxation* is a must. Learning to relax is being kind to your overworked, overworried self. Remember that what you worry about rarely occurs. It's important for you to let go of that tight control over the finances and develop trust in the universe. As a symbolic gesture, buy yourself something elegant and expensive, but also practical, to reinforce your subconscious with the idea that you are financially secure.

Aquarius
Element: Air

NEGATIVE— Know-it-all, rebellious, unreliable, perverse, tactless, disrupting, socially maladapted.
POSITIVE— Insightful, innovative, individualistic, free, independent, truthseeking, reformist, intuitive.

Your self-nurturing highlight is *whatever is different and unusual*. Aquarius Moon thrives on the *outré*—the farther out the better. A natural rebel, it's best for you to satisfy your craving for the different rather than to wait until you build up to the point of running off with a punk rocker! Going against the grain of society is meat and drink to you, but don't overdo this. Even though you may decry anything that seems to want to be in authority over you—including the traditional ways of self-nurturing such as proper meals, sufficient rest, keeping clean and organized, and dressing for the weather—this is actually your key to the freedom you desire. You must learn self-protectiveness by taking care of yourself. Do it your own way—but do it.

Pisces
Element: Water

NEGATIVE— Escapist, addictive, impractical, sentimentalist, illusory, self-sacrificing, self-pitying, guilt-ridden.
POSITIVE— Sensitive, imaginative, sympathetic, artistic, compassionate, aesthetic, subtle, idealistic.

Your self-nurturing highlight is *allowing the spiritual into your life*. When Pisces Moon fails to recognize and provide for its natural connection to the higher realm of Spirit, the results can be drug abuse, alcoholism, depression, even insanity. Pisces Moon needs to be needed and will go to great lengths to contrive this situation. You must recognize that your own needs are not only legitimate but are paramount if you are to survive to help others in the future. So, take time for your spiritual pursuits, of whatever nature. Restore yourself through meditation, prayer, free-form dance, spontaneous art, and music. But learn the basics of self-care. The practical world and its often harsh realities are hard for you, but your spiritual self came packaged in a physical body that needs frequent attention.

A powerful technique for getting in touch with the lunar self is to dialogue with your inner child. We all have a child within, often one who was neglected, abandoned, or abused. By admitting that this inner child—who is actually your basic lunar self—exists and deserves the same care and attention you would give to an actual child in your care, you will get in touch with your lunar needs and be better able to fulfill them. Decide *now* to be your own living Moon mother. Remember, men also need to practice the art of self-nurturance. Picture to yourself the ideal mother, and then be that to yourself. You'll not only avoid lunar burnout, but you'll also have taken a big step toward healing *all* of your life. Begin with the following dialogue with your inner child. The more you become acquainted with this lunar part of yourself, the more you will learn about your real needs. This is a meditation you can use frequently as your relationship with your inner child develops. Once you engage in this process, you may find that your inner child will begin appearing in your dreams.

How to Have a Dialogue with Your Inner Child

Meeting and talking to your inner child is a wonderful way to begin to understand your lunar self. Here is a meditation I devised to help you do this. Prepare yourself in the usual way by getting comfortable and relaxed. Try to take a warm bath first, in scented water. Do this meditation at night, preferably when there is a waxing moon in the sky. Create a hushed and restful atmosphere. If there is moonlight, sit or lie in it. If not, light a white candle. Next, close your eyes and imagine a place where you would like to meet your inner child. Usually this is a room, but it could be a garden or a park or the seashore. Then furnish it however you like; decorate it to suit yourself and its purpose. Once you have done this, invite your child to come forth. The child may be eager to have finally heard from you and come bursting in at once, or she or he may be shy, having been ignored for so long. Be patient. As soon as the child arrives, notice everything about it—age, demeanor, clothing, general appearance. Is it clean and tidy or dirty and messy? Treat him or her as you would any guest on whom you wanted to make a good impression. Be polite, kind, considerate. Invite the child to sit across from you or beside you, giving it a choice. Tell the child that you have come to help and love it, to take care of it, to nurture it. Ask what it needs and wants. And then go out and do that thing for yourself. Repeat this often. Your child will grow and become more communicative, and you will be on your way to forming a wonderful relationship with your lunar self, who will teach you how to nurture yourself in the way that is best for you both.

The Phases of the Moon

The moon passes through what are known as *lunar phases*. After the nights in which we observe the newborn Moon's slim, waxing crescent, her full and glowing face illuminates all. She then returns to the opposite-facing, waning sliver. Her energy moves along with these phases.

The *waxing*, or increasing, Moon brings an energy of *expansion*. This is a positive influence, no matter which sign of the zodiac the Moon occupies at the time of waxing. It is the best time to concentrate on issues of growth or a new beginning of any kind. Whatever is seeded now will grow into fruition later.

When the Moon is *full*, the energy moves toward the completion of what was previously set in motion. The lunar energy is at its strongest and most powerful. You can focus this by using the appropriate meditation and affirmations. As the light of the full Moon eliminates shadows, this is an especially good time to work on conditions with vague symptoms that are difficult to diagnose. In your meditations, ask for identification of the source of the problem in order to determine appropriate treatment.

During the period of the *waning* Moon, the energy moves toward *decreasing* and, finally, at the dark Moon, *eliminating*. This phase is ideal for working with negative issues you want to eliminate from your life, including ill health. Now is the time to practice releasing and letting go. Use the waning phase of the Moon to help you discharge all negativity from your life. Loose it and let it go.

The energies of the Moon change slowly, segueing from one phase into the next. After the night of the dark Moon, for example, the energy of the new Moon slowly increases into the expansive phase that will culminate in the full Moon. The energy of the full Moon begins to build two days before the total fullness is achieved, and it continues in effect for another two days afterward, only somewhat diminished in power as the waning phase takes over. The energy of the waning Moon fades slowly as its visible area decreases.

You can increase your sensitivity to the Moon and to your lunar self by making direct contact. To do this, sit facing the direction of the visible Moon. If you cannot see her, acknowledge her by closing your eyes and imagining the beautiful silver crescent or disk in the dark sky. If possible, position yourself in front of a window or go outside where the rays of the Moon can shine on you. Sit quietly for several minutes until you can feel the Moon's energy contacting you. Imagine her luminosity entering your body, connecting your soul to her as the soul of our planetary system. Feel the magnetic pull of the Moon on your sensitivities and allow yourself to be touched within by her softly glowing light. Let it illuminate your "dark night of the soul," inspiring and uplifting you.

afterword The Serpent's Message

"What, however, about that serpent of Eden, who was not worshipped as the lord of life, but humbled, cursed, and rejected?" What is different about that fellow is simply that his role has been taken from him and given to another, a late arrival in his garden, who was now to be revered in his stead as "the Lord that kills and brings to life" (I Samuel 2:6, Hannah's Song). Serpent gods, however, do not die....

— Joseph Campbell
The Mythic Image

Classical man saw sickness as the effect of a divine action, which could be cured only by another divine action: the divine sickness was to be cast out by a divine remedy. In *Incubation and Modern Psychotherapy*, C. A. Meier says, "The *divina afflictio* then contains its own diagnosis, therapy and prognosis, provided of course that the right attitude toward it is adopted."

At the classical sanctuaries of healing in ancient Greece, a distinctly spiritual atmosphere was created. Dedicated to the god of healing, these ancient "hospitals" had as their primary aim the connecting of the patient with his innermost depths, from where the healing would come. Removed from the distractions and disturbances of the outside world, patients were presented with the opportunity to themselves effect their cure, the elements of which already resided within them. When sickness is vested with such dignity, it has the inestimable advantage of being the agent of its own cure. Thus, what might be termed *spiritual homeopathy* was practiced in the clinics of antiquity, through the medium of dreams and what today we call altered states of consciousness.

Asklepios, the patron god of physicians in ancient Greece carried a plain staff with a single snake coiled around it, and snakes freely roamed his temples. At the Asklepeion, or temple of healing, both patient and doctor made ritual sacrifices, after which the patient retired into seclusion within the temple to await a dream message from the god about his illness and its cure. The mystery of recovery was a private matter between the individual and the god responsible for it. In principle, the physician was excluded from the process.

In *The Mythic Image*, Joseph Campbell elucidates a lovely representation of the dream-cure of the temple sleep:

> In the background is the invalid, dreaming, and at the right his own vision of himself standing, as though having just

emerged in spirit from his ailing body. At the left this figure has advanced to be cured by the god, who is touching his ailing shoulder, while on the couch, simultaneously, the same shoulder is being licked by a snake, which...has emerged from the dreamer himself.

In interpreting the image, Campbell has described an out-of-body experience, many of which have been related by seriously ill or suddenly traumatized people.

Many cultures acknowledge the serpent as representative of the divine power of healing into wholeness, and of rebirth into the spirit, or eternal life.* In this regard, describing a "typical Indian serpent king," at the entrance to a Buddhist temple, in his right hand a burgeoning stalk of the tree of life and in his left a jar of the liquor of immortality, Campbell says:

> [These are] the very gifts that the serpent of Eden had in store for our first parents as the treasure of his second tree....the usual mythological association of the serpent is not, as in the Bible, with corruption, but with physical and spiritual health, as in the Greek caduceus.

Doctors today still use the caduceus as the emblem of their profession.

Such positive serpent images are found from ancient pre-Christian and Asian non-Christian to pre-Columbian Middle America. For example, a fourth-century Roman carving of the patron goddess of health and healing, Hygieia, shows her with a serpent emerging from a sacred vessel and coiling itself about her body. In Mesopotamia, c. 2500 B.C.E., a cylinder seal shows the serpent goddess presiding over the Tree of Life; a

---

*For a full discussion of serpent symbolism, see *The Mythic Image*, pp. 281-300.

fifth-century B.C.E. stone plaque represents the goddess of the Eleusinian mysteries with her symbolic serpents in attendance (the famous oracle of Delphi received illumination from serpents). Vishnu, the sleeping god who heads the Hindu pantheon, rests upon the coils of the abyssal serpent Ananta, the meaning of whose name is "Unending."

Motifs go back as far as 2000 B.C.E. in Sumer and the Indus Valley. An example is the famous cup of King Gudea of Lagash, c. 2000 B.C.E., which is formed of two serpents entwined about an axial rod, adumbrating both kundalini and the caduceus—which belongs to none other than classical Hermes, guide of souls to rebirth in eternal life.

In India, the so-called "serpent power" is a leading motif of yogic symbolism. There, awakening the goddess Kundalini, who is said to be a serpent sleeping coiled at the base of the spine, is the primary task of the yogi embarked on the path of spiritual development. Kundalini is a subtle spiritual force that rises up the spinal column from the lower end to the top of the head, through a system of energy-centers called *chakras*. Activation of the chakras through meditation accelerates health and well-being and confers enlightenment. This remarkable force consists of two strands—one male, one female—which, intertwining, rise through each of the seven chakras in succession, transforming the yogi both psychologically and physically.

Because it sheds its skin in order to grow and renew itself, the serpent is, in non-Christian cultures, the symbol of *rebirth into the spirit*. The Moon is its celestial counterpart—the cycles of waxing and waning, or "dying" (the New Moon), and being reborn (the first crescent sliver) are analogous to the serpent sloughing its skin and being renewed. A scene depicted on a Sumerian seal shows the god enthroned before a caduceus; holding the cup of immortality directly beneath a crescent Moon, he offers a worshipper the drink.

The Serpent's Message

Mythologically, both the serpent and the Moon are symbols of the progress of human life through Time, from the mystery of birth through the mystery of death, to be considered as processes of the same One. Astrologically, the Moon rules bodily functions, and its progressions coincide with the Saturn cycle. A symbol of the Great Mother Goddess—who both gives life and devours the dead—the Moon is related to old Father Time, also known as the Lord of Karma. As such, Saturn—which in alchemical terms equals lead, the *prima materia*, or base matter—symbolizes the restrictions of the temporal universe, of which our bodies are the visible manifestation.

Because each of us carries an archive of all of our experience through life with us—internalized not only in our mind, memories, and emotions, but also in our *bodies*—it is possible to regard the physical body as an expression of both our innate dynamics and our psychology. Our bodies are the record of the fulfillment and deprivation of inward needs.

Exemplifying the necessity to accept the limitations of the physical realm, Saturn is said to be exalted in Libra, the zodiacal sign of balance and harmony. In a harmonious arrangement, be it a work of art or a healthy human, there is an *integration* of the ideal vision with necessary limits: one without the other is disharmony. Power flows when the opposites are united in a harmonious pattern, as is seen in the intertwined snakes of the caduceus and kundalini. Wholeness and health result from integrating *all* aspects of our existence, including sickness and death, which cannot be avoided.

The serpent also represents the psychic realm; when the serpent appears, it signals that the deepest level of the intuitive mind is sending an important message to the conscious mind. An example is one of Jung's patients who, knowing nothing of serpent symbolism, produced a drawing of an eye flanked by two serpents, each "biting" one corner of the eye. Jung remarks of this middle-aged woman that she, "without being neurotic, was struggling for spiritual development and used for this purpose the method of active imagination...to make a drawing of the birth of a new insight."

The symbol of the eye at the center being bitten by the serpents indicates the new ability to "see" the truth of her inner self, to encounter the ultimate and moving power of the universe, transcending and overcoming its pain. Compare this to the "dream-cure" on the ancient Greek tablet described earlier. Such images speak to the deepest mystery of Being, to the unfathomable Nature of ourselves and the universe. These motifs are deeply embedded in our collective unconscious and arise spontaneously when appropriate to the person's psychological and spiritual development.

As an illustration, here is a dream I had while attending the clinic in Bad Bruckenau, which I called *Dream of the Jeweled Serpent*:

> I am given an enormous, beautiful, green serpent, the size of a python. Its intensely-colored iridescent body is set with sparkling gems—rubies, emeralds, sapphires, diamonds, amethysts, garnets, peridots. This glorious creature's eyes are strikingly clear and luminous, like a cat's. Suddenly, it begins thrashing around, spewing excrement. Serpents are an unknown quantity to me, and I haven't the faintest idea how to care for it, nor what is wrong. I phone a friend who is an expert. When I ask what is causing this alarming behavior, she tells me that when serpents are upset, "They shit all over the place." She then says my serpent is upset because *I do not love it*.

The message was clear. Though I had initially come to Bad Bruckenau to recover from physical debilitation, the real problem was much deeper. For several years, I had devoted myself to serving the needs of others. Though I did not regret it,

The Serpent's Message

I realized that—as a result of having totally submerged myself in that endeavor—I had lost the sense of my whole self, not only damaging my health but precipitating an identity crisis. I began to rethink my life to find new direction at a level intrinsic to my SELF. Two months later, I discovered my latent psychic abilities, which served to redirect my life and work. The dream, it seems, presaged this development.

At about this time, also in Bad Bruckenau, I had what seemed an important synchronistic experience. In the courtyard of a nineteenth century Catholic church, I encountered a surprising figure of the Virgin Mary. An uninspired wood carving, she stood on her pedestal in the usual pious pose, hands folded, gazing fondly downward. But she was *not* firmly stamping on the serpent of evil and temptation as usual. Instead, I saw to my astonishment, at eye-level from the ground where I stood, that the serpent was curled cozily around her bare feet as the *oroborus* (serpent biting its tail), a symbol of wholeness and the regeneration of life. I could not help but wonder if the artist were aware of the symbolism and meant it as a covert reference, or if this amazing representation stemmed from his unconscious depths.

Healing methods of indigenous peoples are generally gathered under the general term of *shamanism*, which is the religion of many traditional cultures throughout the world. Originating in central and northern Asia, it spread outward—into the New World, Australia, Africa, and other parts of Asia. Shamanism speaks directly to the totality that encompasses all life and the environment, both terrestrial and celestial, in which that life resides and has its being. There is no separation of spirit and body, of human and animal/plant, of earth and cosmos.

In these cultures, too, the serpent motif abounds. In Mexico, Quetzalcoatl, The Lord of Life and Death (whose symbol is the cross and whose mother was a virgin), is known as "The Plumed Serpent." The Mayan god Kukulcan, like Christ, sloughs off death to be resurrected. An early stone carving depicts him as "The Feathered Serpent"—an ornately elegant snake rising up on its own coils to tower over a worshipper holding an offering. And, in a pre-Columbian Aztec altar design, two snakes are intertwined into a perfect caduceus form, their heads facing in opposite directions.

Among numerous North American designs, one engraved shell depicts a pair of ornamented serpent dancers emerging from a rattlesnake skin, their tails intertwined into a caduceus-like shape. Campbell says of this image that the serpent dancers "reiterate the universal serpent-theme of renewal of life through the sloughing of death."

The basic tenet of this worldview is that life exists simultaneously in two realms—the everyday or "natural" one and the transpersonal, or spiritual, one. Analogous to the "Gaia principle," proposed by J. Lovelock in 1979, which states that Earth is a living, breathing organism, this idea of an alive, organic Earth—now gradually taking hold upon our collective consciousness—is at the base of shamanism. What I call "the invisible world" is recognized by these cultures as being every bit as important as, and even more potent than, the manifest, or visible, world. In shamanism, the realm of the spirit is considered to be both antecedent to and continuing after the visible forms it brings into being. In these traditional societies, the spiritual aspect of life always takes precedence over the merely physical or bodily realities. As Emanuel Swedenborg, the eighteenth-century scientist-turned-visionary who developed a theory of "correspondences," said, "There is nothing in nature that does not symbolize something in the world of spirit."

Traditionally, tribal shamans have nurtured spiritual powers and brought them to a high degree of development, passing their knowledge and techniques along to succeeding generations. Wise in the lore of herbs and plants known to have

The Serpent's Message

healing properties, the shaman fuses the practice of spiritual magic with the practice of healing. Indeed, there is no separation between the two—the practice of shamanism presupposes that we live in a psychospiritual as well as physical ecosystem. In this view, the entire world and all in it are imbued with spirit—all life is in communication at a deep level, beneath our awareness. Animals have their own type of consciousness and can know our thoughts and sense our feelings (as anyone with a pet cat or dog can attest).

Today, leading edge scientists such as physicist David Foster and Cambridge University biologist Rupert Sheldrake postulate natural, if unseen, forces that possess both intelligence and purpose. Sheldrake's concept of "morphic fields," in which there is a consistent if invisible communion between all members of a species, is similar to the shamanistic idea of an archetypal or "master" animal for each species.

Shamans believe they can transcend both time and space and, in so doing, avail themselves of the invisible powers, which reside in the animal and vegetable kingdoms and in the elements—fire, earth, air, water. Alchemy, like the magic of the shamans, was the attempt to make contact with invisible energy sources.

It is sad that in our society the correspondences between religion, magic, and medicine have been all but lost. Members of the medical establishment, in their search for power over Nature, have fallen prey to the negative aspects of Saturn—narrowing and restricting their view to the physical body and the material aspects of illness, health, and life itself. Thus, they are prevented from practicing the healing magic of the serpent god. Though they display the wand of Hermes on their license plates, they have lost the sense of the living symbol of their craft. This is because they do not—or will not—see that nonphysical forces are what animate and support the manifest world, including that of the physical body.

Healing Mind, Body, Spirit

The contributions of science to our health are important and valuable, but the mind-set of the medical community does not allow for the interplay of all the energies of mind, body, and spirit. We ourselves must be responsible for recognizing our need for wholeness and integrating it into our lives. The necessity for healing—not only of ourselves but also of our societies and our planet—is immediate, one might say *urgent*. We cannot wait for those who do not grasp the concept of wholeness, which lies at the root of all healing and health, to give us permission to explore our own natures and use them fully. We must, as Nietzsche says, "Live as though the day were here."

By so doing, we incorporate the divine serpent power into our daily lives and enable ourselves to make far-reaching changes both in ourselves and in our society. My dream is that one day many gentle and caring places of healing, where the necessary transformational processes will be honored, encouraged, and nurtured, will replace a health-care *industry* that, for profit, serves up hurried and impersonal care to the sick and dying. I envision a time when enlightened healers, while being adequately paid for their services, will come to the work as to a sacred calling.

Assuming order and meaning in all the balance-seeking processes of the SELF, it is possible to view illness and healing as permutations of the life pulse. Both can be seen as a fundamental *rebalancing* of our inner order with that of the natural order. As the *Matri Upanishad* tells us, "The course of the inner Self is measured by the course of the outer Self . . . and the course of the outer Self is measured by the course of the inner Self . . . within the lotus of the heart."

Each day we have the opportunity to *recreate* ourselves by tuning into the SELF in ourselves and in the All. When we activate our energies in the form of impulses and desires; when we seek out both our strengths and our weaknesses fearlessly; when we test our abilities anew with the challenges life presents; we then develop into the unique individuals we came into this world to be.

But when we hesitate, hold back, and court fear instead of trust, we stultify our essential life energies. Because the psyche persists in realizing what one is innately meant to be, when the *quality* of our lives becomes less than we inherently know it should be, warning bells sound in the form of physical illness and psychological distress. Crisis arises to command our attention to what is wrong, forcing buried issues into the light where we can attend to our need for healing. In support of this point, here are some observations made by Edward C. Whitmont in his book *The Alchemy of Healing*:

> [In] the human healing process the entelechy may be expected to guide transformation....It may, therefore, even be bent upon imbalancing and upsetting an existing state of health if and when this state no longer accords with the growth needs of the personality...growth may call for wounding or partial destruction [as] expressed by the Delphic Oracle of Apollo that "that which wounds shall also heal."

And, as we act to heal ourselves by allowing our entelechy to guide us, we heal others and the environments in which we live—family, community, the species, the planet.

True, there is much that is negative in our world—as the TV newscast nightly confirms—and in our individual lives, which are often beset by ill health and emotional pain. But I am one who firmly believes that it is better to light a candle than to curse the darkness. One lighted candle can serve to light millions of other candles—can, ultimately, create a blaze of light that will illuminate the entire world.

Healing Mind, Body, Spirit

We do not just receive the fire of life and pass it on unchanged, like an Olympic torch relay runner. In bearing that living flame, we add that which is uniquely our own to its power and glory. Life is a vast ecosystem in which we all play our parts—just as does each rock and plant, bird and bee—and every individual contribution is of vital importance. Our lives are not just to continue human existence—each of us has the potential to add to the quality of life itself, to increase the sum total of positive energy in the world. For myself, I know that the closer I get to expressing the reality of who I am, the more healed and whole I become. It is in this spirit that I bring you the serpent's message. I believe that we owe it both to ourselves and to the totality of life on Earth to heed its wisdom.

appendix one
Selected Bibliography

Abadie, M. J. *Your Psychic Potential*. Holbrook, MA: Adams Media Corp., 1995.

Achterberg, Jeanne. *Imagery in Healing: Shamanism and Modern Medicine*. Boston: New Science Library, 1985.

—. *Woman as Healer*. Boston: Shambhala, 1991.

Anderson-Evangelista, Anita. *Hypnosis: A Journey into the Mind*. New York: Arco, 1980.

Bandler, Richard, and John Grinder. *Using Your Brain—For a Change*. Moab, UT: Real People Press, 1985.

Beck, A. T. *Cognitive Therapy and Emotional Disorders*. New York: International Universities Press, 1976.

Bennett, Hal Zina. *Inner Guides, Visions, Dreams, and Dr. Einstein*. Berkeley, CA: Celestial Arts, 1986.

Benson, Herbert. *The Relaxation Response*. New York: Avon, 1975.

—. *The Mind/Body Effect*. New York: Simon & Schuster, 1979.

Bohm, David. *Wholeness and the Implicate Order*. Boston: Ark Paperbacks, 1980.

Bohm, David, and F. David Peat. *Science, Order, and Creativity*. New York: Bantam, 1980.

Borysenko, Joan. *Minding the Body, Mending the Mind*. Reading, MA: Addison-Wesley, 1987.

Brown, Joseph Epes. *The Spiritual Legacy of the American Indian*. New York: Crossroad Publishing Co., 1982.

Bry, Adelaide, and Marjorie Bair. *Directing the Movies of the Mind: Visualization for Health and Insight*. New York: Harper & Row, 1978.

Campbell, Joseph. Assisted by M. J. Abadie. *The Mythic Image*. Princeton, NJ: Princeton University Press, 1974.

—. *The Hero with a Thousand Faces*. New York: Bollingen Foundation, 1961.

—. *Occidental Mythology*. Vol. 2, *The Masks of God*. New York: Viking Press, 1964.

—. *Creative Mythology*. Vol. 4, *The Masks of God*. New York: Viking Press, 1965.

Caudill, M. *Managing Pain Before It Manages You*. New York: Guilford Press, 1994.

Cunningham, Donna. *Moon Signs*. New York: Ballantine, 1988.

—. *Healing Pluto Problems*. York Beach, ME: Samuel Weiser, 1986.

Dickenson, Emily. *Selected Poems and Letters of Emily Dickenson*. Edited by Robert N. Linscott. New York: Doubleday-Anchor, 1959.

Domar, Alice D., and Henry Dreher. *Healing Mind, Healthy Woman*. New York: Henry Holt, 1996.

Dossey, Larry. *Space, Time and Medicine*. Boston: Shambhala Publications, 1982.

—. *Meaning and Medicine*. New York: Bantam Books, 1991.

Geddes, Sheila. *Astrology and Health*. London: Foulsham, 1992.

George, Demetra. *Mysteries of the Dark Moon*. San Francisco: Harper San Francisco, 1992.

George, Leonard. *The Silent Pulse: A Search for the Perfect Rhythm that Exists in Each of Us*. New York: Bantam, 1978.

Selected Bibliography

Greene, Liz. "Alchemical Symbolism in the Horoscope." In *Dynamics of the Unconscious*. York Beach, ME: Samuel Weiser, 1988.

Grossinger, Richard. *Planet Medicine: From Stone Age Shamanism to Post-Industrial Healing*. Berkeley, CA: North Atlantic Books, 1987.

Hall, Nor. *The Moon and the Virgin*. New York: Harper Colophon Books, 1980.

Heisenberg, Werner. *Physics and Philosophy: The Revolution in Modern Science*. New York: Harper, 1971.

Jung, Carl. *Alchemical Studies*. Vol. 13, *The Collected Works of C. G. Jung*. Bollingen Series XX. Princeton, NJ: Princeton University Press, 1968.

—. *Psychology and Alchemy*. Vol. 12, *The Collected Works of C. G. Jung*. Bollingen Series XX. Princeton, NJ: Princeton University Press, 1968.

—. *The Development of Personality*. Vol. 17, *The Collected Works of C. G. Jung*. New York: Pantheon Books, 1954.

Kerenyi, Carl, *Asklepios: Archetypal Image of the Physician's Existence*. Translated by Ralph Manheim. New York: Bollingen Series, Pantheon Books, 1959.

Kreinheder, Albert. *Body and Soul: The Other Side of Illness*. Toronto: Inner City Books, 1991.

Larsen, Stephen. *The Mythic Imagination*. New York: Bantam, 1992.

—. *The Shaman's Doorway*. New York: Harper & Row, 1976.

LeShan, Lawrence. *Cancer as a Turning Point*. New York: Dutton Books, 1989.

Levi, Primo. *The Drowned and the Saved*. New York: Summit Books, 1988.

Levine, Stephen. *Healing into Life and Death*. Garden City, NJ: Anchor Books/Doubleday, 1987.

Locke, Steven, and Douglas Colligan. *The Healer Within: The New Medicine of Mind and Body*. New York: E. P. Dutton, 1986.

Lorde, Audre. *A Burst of Light*. Ithaca, NY: Firebrand Books, 1988.

Mindell, Arnold. *Working with the Dreaming Body*. Boston: Routledge & Kegan Paul, 1985.

Montagu, A. *Touching: The Human Significance of the Skin*. New York: Harper & Row, 1978.

Monte, Tom, and Editors of EastWest Natural Health. *World Medicine: The East West Guide to Healing Your Body*. New York: G. P. Putnam's Sons, 1963.

Moss, Howard, *Finding Them Lost*. New York: Charles Scribners & Sons, 1965.

Neumann. *Art and the Creative Unconscious*, Bollingen Series LXI. Princeton, NJ: Princeton University Press, 1971.

—. *The Great Mother*. Bollingen Series XLVII. New York: Pantheon Books, 1955.

Northrup, C. *Women's Bodies, Women's Wisdom: Creating Physical and Emotional Health and Healing*. New York: Bantam Books, 1994.

Ornstein, R., and D. Sobel. *Healthy Pleasures*. Reading, MA: Addison-Wesley, 1989.

Paracelsus. *Selected Writings*. Edited by Jolande Jacobi. Translated by Norbert Guterman. Princeton, NJ: Princeton University Press, 1951.

Pelletier, Kenneth. *Mind as Healer, Mind as Slayer*. New York: Dell Books, 1977.

Pennebaker, J. W. *Opening Up: The Healing Power of Confiding in Others*. New York: William Morrow and Co., 1990.

Perera, Sylvia Brinton. *Descent to the Goddess*. Toronto: Inner City Books, 1981.

Ponce, Charles. *Alchemy*. Berkeley, CA: North Atlantic Books, 1983.

Ponder, Catharine. *The Dynamic Laws of Healing*. Marina del Rey, CA: De Vorss, 1985.

Rodin, J. *Body Traps: Breaking the Binds that Keep You from Feeling Good about Your Body*. New York: William Morrow and Co., 1992.

Sheldrake, Rupert. *The Rebirth of Nature*. Rochester, VT: Park Street Press, 1991.

Temoshok, L., and H. Dreher. *The Type C Connection: The Behavioral Links to Cancer and Your Health*. New York: Random House, 1992.

Weil, Andrew. *Health and Healing*. Boston: Houghton Mifflin, 1985.

Whitmont, Edward C. *The Symbolic Quest*. Princeton, NJ: Princeton University Press, 1991.

—. *The Alchemy of Healing*. Berkeley, CA: North Atlantic Books, 1993.

Wickes, Frances. *The Inner World of Choice*. New York: Harper and Row, 1963.

—. *The Inner World of Childhood*. New York: Appleton-Century-Crofts, Inc., 1927.

appendix two
Resources

~ Flower Remedies

Where to purchase flower remedies:

Bach Flower Remedies can be obtained from Nelson Bach, 1007 West Upsal St., Philadelphia, PA 19119, 1-800-314-BACH, which is the American source for the original Bach Flower Remedies made in England. They also carry a line of homeopathic products. Excellent service.

Ellon Company, Box 320, Woodmere, NY 11598 carries a line of flower remedies. They follow the original Bach formulas but are made in the United States.

California remedies are available from Flower Essence Services, Box 586, Nevada City, CA 94939.

Other remedies can be had from Pegasus Products, Inc., Box 228, Boulder, CO 80306.

Books about flower remedies:

Bach, Edward, M.D. and F. J. Wheeler, M.D., *The Bach Flower Remedies*, Keats Health Books, New Canaan, CT, 1979.

Healing Mind, Body, Spirit

Considered to be the "bible" on the Bach Flower Remedies, this book is written by the man who developed them. However, the book listed next is both more comprehensible and comprehensive.

Chancellor, Dr. Phillip M., *Handbook of the Bach Flower Remedies*, Keats Health Books, New Canaan, CT, 1971.

This is the book I recommend most for anyone wanting to learn the Remedies. Keyword descriptions of the Remedies are followed by complete descriptions of the personality traits to which each is applicable. Numerous case histories detail the Remedies used for specific conditions, and the physical ailments that were healed as a result.

The Flower Essence Journal, Flower Essence Services, Box 586, Nevada City, CA 94939, is a periodical/newsletter covering flower essences and their uses.

Healing-Related Publications

The Institute of Noetic Sciences, 475 Gate 5 Rd., Sausalito, CA 94965, publishes a quarterly journal that explores issues of mind/body and consciousness. Highly recommended.

Advances is a quarterly journal published by *The Journal of Mind-Body Health*, P.O. Box 3000, Denville NY 07834. It contains mind/body literature drawn from numerous journals and original articles.

"Brain/Mind Bulletin," P.O. Box 42211, Los Angeles, CA 90042, is published by Marilyn Ferguson, author of *The Aquarian Conspiracy*. It is an update on research covering mind/body medicine, physics, and consciousness. The American Holistic Medicine Association publishes a quarterly journal, *Holistic Medicine*, that features readable articles on the entire span of alternative, or complementary, medicines.

Common Boundary, P.O. Box 445, Mt. Morris, IL 61054, is a bi-monthly magazine that explores the boundary between psychology and spirituality. It gives comprehensive listings of

Resources

conferences and programs being held throughout the country in mind/body medicine and psychology.

Spindrift Inc., Century Plaza Building, 100 W. Main St., Suite 408, Lansdale, PA 19446, a not-for-profit corporation "chartered for the purpose of education and research in spiritual healing," publishes a quarterly newsletter.

Holistic Health Directory, New Age Journal Publications, 342 Western Avenue, Brighton, MA 02135, is a comprehensive guide that lists clinics specializing in mind/body medicine, homeopathy, and various other alternative methods.

The Self-Help Sourcebook, published by American Self-Help Clearing House, St. Clares-Riverside Medical Center, 25 Pocono Rd., Denville NJ 07834, is a comprehensive resource for finding and forming mutual aid self-help groups.

The Fetzer Institute, 9292 West KL Ave., Kalamazoo, MI 49009, publishes Advances: *The Journal of Mind-Body Health*.

Organizations and Medical Resources

American Holistic Health Association, P.O. Box 17400, Anaheim, CA, is an educational, nonprofit association that offers free literature and resources for healing.

The National Center for Homeopathy will refer physicians who use homeopathic methods. Call (703) 548-7790 for information.

Homeopathic Educational Services, 2124 Kittredge St., Berkeley, CA 94704, is a mail order and retail company that provides books, tapes, remedies, and information about homeopathic resources worldwide.

Write the American Chiropractic Association, 1701 Clarendon Blvd., Arlington, VA 22209 for information on the names of practitioners in your area.

For information on acupuncture, and a list of medical doctors who use it, contact the American Academy of Medical

Acupuncture, 5820 Wilshire Blvd., Suite 500, Los Angeles, CA 90036.

NALPRALERT (Natural Products Alert), College of Pharmacy-UIC, 833 S. Wood St., Chicago, IL, has a database of 126,000 published articles on specific herbal products. A fee of 75 cents per reference is charged.

The American Association of Naturopathic Physicians (AANP), 2366 Eastlake Ave. E, Suite 322, Seattle, WA 98102, is the leading professional organization. It publishes the *Journal of Naturopathic Medicine* and maintains a list to help locate local naturopathic physicians.

The American Chronic Pain Association, P.O. Box 850, Rocklin, CA 95677, manages a list of over 500 support groups internationally; it also publishes workbooks and a newsletter.

The Center for Attitudinal Healing, 33 Buchanan, Sausalito, CA 94965, has support groups throughout the nation for people with chronic or life-threatening illness.

The Wellness Community, 2716 Ocean Park Blvd., Suite 1040, Santa Monica, CA 90405 provides a similar service and also offers audiotape programs in mind/body medicine.

The Nurse Healers Professional Associates, Inc., P.O. Box 444, Allison Park, PA 15101, provides information about Therapeutic Touch and training.

The American Academy of Reflexology, 606 E. Magnolia Blvd., Suite B, Burbank, CA 91501, can provide referrals to certified practitioners.

The Mind/Body Medical Institute, Division of Behavioral Medicine, Deaconess Hospital, 1 Deaconess Road, Boston, MA 02215, is headed by Herbert Benson, M.D. Write to them for a list of affiliates and information about tapes they sell.

Hay House, Inc., 1154 E. Dominguez St., P.O. Box 6204, Carson, CA 90749-6204, maintains a listing of therapists and spiritual healers throughout the country. Information is free and can be accessed by zip code.

The Hoffman Institute, 14 Scenic Ave., San Anselmo, CA 94960, offers a week-long residential program based on a psychospiritual model for healing the wounds of childhood, transforming old patterns, and learning forgiveness (especially for one's parents).

Women to Women, One Pleasant St., Yarmouth, ME 04096, Dr. Christiane Northrup's Center for Women's Health, places a strong emphasis on holistic and mind-body medicine.

For eating disorders, contact National Eating Disorders Organization, 445 East Granville Rd., Worthington, OH 43085 or American Anorexia/Bulimia Association, 418 East 76th St., New York, NY 10021. Overeaters Anonymous, Inc. has a world service office at P.O. Box 44020, Rio Rancho, NM 87174.

appendix three
Moon Ephemeris: How to Find Your Moon Sign

Find the year of birth in the tables provided. Then find the birth month at the top of the tables. Find date of birth in the column below it. If it is not listed, then the sign listed for the earlier date is the Moon sign. For instance, if you were born on February 3, 1950, you would see that for February 2, the sign listed is Leo, meaning the moon was in the sign Leo. For February 5, Virgo is listed. This means that the moon is in the sign Leo until February 5 and your Moon is in the sign Leo.

If you are born on a day that starts a new sign (February 5 in this example), your Moon may be in the preceding sign. The only way to be absolutely sure is to have your chart done professionally or by a computer service. In lieu of this, read the text for both signs, and see which seems more like you.

1950

JAN	FEB	MAR	APR	MAY	JUN	JUL	AUG	SEP	OCT	NOV	DEC
1 GEM	1 CAN	1 CAN	1 VIR	1 LIB	1 SAG	1 CAP	1 PIS	1 ARI	1 GEM	1 CAN	1 LEO
4 CAN	2 LEO	2 LEO	3 LIB	2 SCO	2 AQU	2 ARI	2 TAU	4 CAN	3 LEO	2 VIR
6 LEO	5 VIR	4 VIR	5 SCO	4 SAG	4 AQU	4 PIS	5 TAU	4 GEM	6 LEO	5 VIR	5 LIB
8 VIR	7 LIB	6 LIB	7 SAG	6 CAP	7 PIS	6 ARI	8 GEM	7 CAN	9 VIR	7 LIB	7 SCO
10 LIB	9 SCO	8 SCO	9 CAP	8 AQU	9 ARI	9 TAU	10 CAN	9 LEO	11 LIB	9 SCO	9 SAG
13 SCO	11 SAG	10 SAG	11 AQU	10 PIS	12 TAU	11 GEM	13 LEO	11 VIR	13 SCO	11 SAG	11 CAP
15 SAG	13 CAP	12 CAP	13 PIS	13 ARI	14 GEM	14 CAN	15 VIR	13 LIB	15 SAG	13 CAP	13 AQU
17 CAP	15 AQU	15 AQU	16 ARI	15 TAU	17 CAN	16 LEO	17 LIB	16 SCO	17 CAP	15 AQU	15 PIS
19 AQU	18 PIS	17 PIS	18 TAU	18 GEM	19 LEO	19 VIR	19 SCO	18 SAG	19 AQU	18 PIS	17 ARI
21 PIS	20 ARI	19 ARI	21 GEM	20 CAN	21 VIR	21 LIB	21 SAG	20 CAP	21 PIS	20 ARI	20 TAU
24 ARI	23 TAU	22 TAU	23 CAN	23 LEO	23 LIB	23 SCO	23 CAP	22 AQU	24 ARI	22 TAU	22 GEM
26 TAU	25 GEM	24 GEM	26 LEO	25 VIR	26 SCO	25 SAG	26 AQU	24 PIS	26 TAU	25 GEM	25 CAN
29 GEM	28 CAN	27 CAN	28 VIR	28 LIB	28 SAG	28 CAP	28 PIS	26 ARI	29 GEM	28 CAN	27 LEO
31 CAN		29 LEO	30 LIB	29 SCO	30 CAP	29 AQU	30 ARI	29 TAU	31 CAN	30 LEO	30 VIR
		31 VIR		31 SAG		31 PIS	31 ARI				31 VIR

1951

JAN	FEB	MAR	APR	MAY	JUN	JUL	AUG	SEP	OCT	NOV	DEC
1 LIB	1 SCO	1 SAG	1 AQU	1 ARI	1 ARI	1 GEM	1 CAN	1 VIR	1 LIB	1 SCO	1 CAP
3 SCO	2 SAG	3 CAP	3 PIS	3 ARI	2 TAU	4 CAN	3 LEO	4 LIB	3 SCO	2 SAG	3 AQU
5 SAG	4 CAP	5 AQU	6 ARI	5 TAU	4 GEM	6 LEO	5 VIR	6 SCO	5 SAG	4 CAP	5 PIS
7 CAP	6 AQU	7 PIS	8 TAU	8 GEM	7 CAN	9 VIR	7 LIB	8 SAG	8 CAP	6 AQU	7 ARI
9 AQU	8 PIS	9 ARI	11 GEM	10 CAN	9 LEO	11 LIB	10 SCO	10 CAP	10 AQU	8 PIS	10 TAU
11 PIS	10 ARI	12 TAU	13 CAN	13 LEO	12 VIR	14 SCO	12 SAG	12 AQU	12 PIS	10 ARI	12 GEM
14 ARI	12 TAU	14 GEM	16 LEO	15 VIR	14 LIB	16 SAG	14 CAP	14 PIS	14 ARI	13 TAU	15 CAN
16 TAU	15 GEM	17 CAN	18 VIR	18 LIB	16 SCO	18 CAP	16 AQU	17 ARI	17 TAU	15 GEM	17 LEO
19 GEM	17 CAN	19 LEO	20 LIB	20 SCO	18 SAG	20 AQU	18 PIS	19 TAU	19 GEM	17 CAN	20 VIR
21 CAN	20 LEO	22 VIR	22 SCO	22 SAG	20 CAP	22 PIS	20 ARI	21 GEM	21 CAN	20 LEO	22 LIB
24 LEO	22 VIR	24 LIB	24 SAG	24 CAP	22 AQU	24 ARI	22 TAU	24 CAN	24 LEO	22 VIR	24 SCO
26 VIR	24 LIB	26 SCO	26 AQU	26 AQU	24 PIS	26 TAU	25 GEM	26 LEO	26 VIR	25 LIB	27 SAG
28 LIB	27 SCO	28 SAG	28 AQU	28 PIS	26 ARI	29 GEM	27 CAN	29 VIR	28 LIB	27 SCO	29 CAP
30 SCO	28 SCO	30 CAP	30 AQU	30 ARI	29 TAU	31 CAN	30 LEO	30 VIR	31 SCO	29 SAG	31 AQU
31 SCO		31 CAP		31 ARI	30 TAU		31 LEO			30 SAG	

1952

JAN	FEB	MAR	APR	MAY	JUN	JUL	AUG	SEP	OCT	NOV	DEC
1 AQU	1 ARI	1 TAU	1 GEM	1 CAN	1 VIR	1 LIB	1 SAG	1 CAP	1 PIS	1 ARI	1 GEM
2 PIS	2 TAU	3 GEM	2 CAN	2 LEO	3 LIB	3 SCO	3 CAP	2 AQU	3 ARI	2 TAU	4 CAN
4 ARI	5 GEM	5 CAN	4 LEO	4 VIR	5 SCO	5 SAG	5 AQU	4 PIS	5 TAU	4 GEM	6 LEO
6 TAU	7 CAN	8 LEO	7 VIR	7 LIB	8 SAG	7 CAP	7 PIS	6 ARI	8 GEM	6 CAN	8 GEM
8 GEM	10 LEO	11 VIR	9 LIB	9 SCO	10 CAP	9 AQU	9 ARI	8 TAU	10 CAN	9 LEO	11 LIB
11 CAN	12 VIR	13 LIB	12 SCO	11 SAG	12 AQU	12 PIS	12 TAU	10 GEM	12 LEO	11 VIR	14 SCO
13 LEO	15 LIB	15 SCO	14 SAG	13 CAP	14 PIS	14 ARI	14 GEM	13 CAN	15 VIR	14 LIB	16 SAG
16 VIR	17 SCO	18 SAG	16 CAP	15 AQU	16 ARI	16 TAU	16 CAN	15 LEO	17 LIB	16 SCO	18 CAP
18 LIB	19 SAG	20 CAP	18 AQU	17 PIS	18 TAU	18 GEM	19 LEO	18 VIR	20 SCO	18 SAG	20 AQU
21 SCO	21 CAP	22 AQU	20 PIS	20 ARI	20 GEM	20 CAN	21 VIR	21 LIB	22 SAG	21 CAP	22 PIS
23 SAG	23 AQU	24 PIS	22 ARI	22 TAU	23 CAN	23 LEO	24 LIB	23 SCO	24 CAP	23 AQU	24 ARI
25 CAP	26 PIS	26 ARI	25 TAU	24 GEM	25 LEO	25 VIR	26 SCO	25 SAG	26 AQU	25 PIS	26 TAU
27 AQU	28 ARI	28 TAU	27 GEM	27 CAN	28 VIR	28 LIB	29 SAG	27 CAP	29 PIS	27 ARI	29 GEM
29 PIS	29 ARI	30 GEM	29 CAN	29 LEO	30 LIB	30 SCO	31 CAP	29 AQU	31 ARI	29 TAU	31 CAN
31 ARI		31 GEM	30 CAN	31 LEO		31 SCO		30 AQU		30 TAU	

241

Healing Mind, Body, Spirit

1953

JAN	FEB	MAR	APR	MAY	JUN	JUL	AUG	SEP	OCT	NOV	DEC
1 CAN	1 VIR	1 VIR	1 LIB	1 SAG	1 CAP	1 AQU	1 ARI	1 GEM	1 CAN	1 VIR	1 LIB
2 LEO	4 LIB	3 LIB	2 SCO	4 CAP	2 AQU	2 PIS	2 TAU	3 CAN	2 LEO	4 LIB	3 SCO
5 VIR	6 SCO	5 SCO	5 SAG	6 AQU	4 PIS	4 ARI	4 GEM	5 LEO	5 VIR	6 SCO	6 SAG
7 LIB	9 SAG	8 SAG	6 CAP	8 PIS	6 ARI	6 TAU	6 CAN	8 VIR	7 LIB	9 SAG	8 CAP
10 SCO	11 CAP	10 CAP	9 AQU	10 ARI	8 TAU	9 GEM	9 LEO	10 LIB	10 SCO	11 CAP	10 AQU
12 SAG	13 AQU	12 AQU	11 PIS	12 TAU	11 GEM	11 CAN	11 VIR	13 SCO	12 SAG	13 AQU	13 PIS
14 CAP	15 PIS	14 F15	13 ARI	14 GEM	13 CAN	13 LEO	14 LIB	15 SAG	15 CAP	15 PIS	15 ARI
15 AQU	17 ARI	16 ARI	15 TAU	16 CAN	15 LEO	15 VIR	16 SCO	17 CAP	17 AQU	18 ARI	17 TAU
18 PIS	19 TAU	18 TAU	17 GEM	19 LEO	18 VIR	18 LIB	19 SAG	19 PIS	19 ARI	20 TAU	19 GEM
20 ARI	21 GEM	20 GEM	19 CAN	21 VIR	20 LIB	20 SCO	21 CAP	22 PIS	21 ARI	22 GEM	21 CAN
23 TAU	23 CAN	23 CAN	21 LEO	24 LIB	23 SCO	22 SAG	23 AQU	24 ARI	23 TAU	24 CAN	23 LEO
25 GEM	26 LEO	25 LEO	24 VIR	26 SCO	25 SAG	25 CAP	25 PIS	26 TAU	25 GEM	26 LEO	26 VIR
27 CAN	28 VIR	28 VIR	27 LIB	29 SAG	27 CAP	27 AQU	27 ARI	28 GEM	27 CAN	28 VIR	28 LIB
30 LEO		30 LIB	29 SCO	31 CAP	29 AQU	29 PIS	29 TAU	30 CAN	30 LEO	30 VIR	31 SCO
31 LEO		31 LIB	30 SCO		30 AQU	31 ARI	31 GEM				

1954

JAN	FEB	MAR	APR	MAY	JUN	JUL	AUG	SEP	OCT	NOV	DEC
1 SCO	1 CAP	1 CAP	1 PIS	1 ARI	1 GEM	1 CAN	1 VIR	1 LIB	1 SCO	1 CAP	1 AQU
2 SAG	3 AQU	3 AQU	3 ARI	3 TAU	3 CAN	3 LEO	4 LIB	2 SCO	2 SAG	4 AQU	3 PIS
5 CAP	5 PIS	5 PIS	5 TAU	5 GEM	5 LEO	5 VIR	6 SCO	5 SAG	5 CAP	6 PIS	5 ARI
7 AQU	7 ARI	7 ARI	7 GEM	7 CAN	8 VIR	7 LIB	9 SAG	7 CAP	7 AQU	8 ARI	7 TAU
9 PIS	9 TAU	9 TAU	9 CAN	9 LEO	10 LIB	10 SCO	11 CAP	10 AQU	9 PIS	10 TAU	9 GEM
11 ARI	11 GEM	11 GEM	12 LEO	11 VIR	12 SCO	12 SAG	13 AQU	12 PIS	11 ARI	12 GEM	11 CAN
13 TAU	14 CAN	13 CAN	14 VIR	14 LIB	15 SAG	14 CAP	15 PIS	14 ARI	13 TAU	14 CAN	13 LEO
15 GEM	16 LEO	15 LEO	16 LIB	16 SCO	17 CAP	17 AQU	18 ARI	16 TAU	15 GEM	16 LEO	16 VIR
17 CAN	18 VIR	18 VIR	19 SCO	19 SAG	19 AQU	19 PIS	20 TAU	18 GEM	18 CAN	19 VIR	18 LIB
20 LEO	21 LIB	20 LIB	21 SAG	21 CAP	22 PIS	21 ARI	22 GEM	20 CAN	20 LEO	21 LIB	21 SCO
22 VIR	23 SCO	23 SCO	23 CAP	24 AQU	24 ARI	24 TAU	24 CAN	23 VIR	22 VIR	23 SCO	23 SAG
25 LIB	26 SAG	25 SAG	26 AQU	26 PIS	26 TAU	26 GEM	26 LEO	25 LIB	25 LIB	26 SAG	26 CAP
27 SCO	28 CAP	28 CAP	28 PIS	28 ARI	28 GEM	28 CAN	29 VIR	27 SCO	27 SCO	28 CAP	28 AQU
30 SAG		30 AQU	30 PIS	30 TAU	30 CAN	30 LEO	31 LIB	30 SAG	30 SAG	30 CAP	30 PIS
31 SAG				31 TAU		31 LEO			31 SAG		31 PIS

1955

JAN	FEB	MAR	APR	MAY	JUN	JUL	AUG	SEP	OCT	NOV	DEC
1 PIS	1 TAU	1 GEM	1 CAN	1 VIR	1 LIB	1 SCO	1 CAP	1 AQU	1 PIS	1 TAU	1 GEM
2 ARI	2 GEM	3 CAN	2 LEO	4 LIB	2 SCO	2 SAG	3 AQU	2 PIS	2 ARI	2 GEM	2 CAN
4 TAU	4 CAN	6 LEO	4 VIR	6 SCO	5 SAG	5 CAP	6 PIS	4 ARI	4 TAU	4 CAN	4 LEO
6 GEM	6 LEO	8 VIR	6 LIB	9 SAG	7 CAP	7 AQU	8 ARI	7 TAU	6 GEM	6 LEO	6 VIR
8 CAN	8 VIR	10 LIB	9 SCO	11 CAP	10 AQU	10 PIS	10 TAU	9 GEM	8 CAN	9 VIR	8 LIB
10 LEO	11 LIB	13 SCO	11 SAG	14 AQU	12 PIS	12 ARI	12 GEM	11 CAN	10 LEO	11 LIB	10 SCO
12 VIR	13 SCO	15 SAG	14 CAP	16 PIS	15 ARI	15 TAU	15 CAN	13 LEO	12 LEO	13 SCO	13 SAG
14 LIB	16 SAG	18 CAP	16 AQU	18 ARI	17 TAU	16 GEM	17 LEO	15 VIR	15 LIB	16 SAG	16 CAP
17 SCO	18 CAP	20 AQU	19 PIS	20 TAU	19 GEM	19 CAN	19 VIR	17 LIB	17 SCO	18 CAP	18 AQU
19 SAG	21 AQU	22 PIS	21 ARI	22 GEM	21 CAN	20 LEO	21 LIB	20 SCO	19 SAG	21 AQU	21 PIS
22 CAP	23 PIS	24 ARI	24 CAN	24 CAN	23 LEO	23 VIR	25 SCO	22 SAG	22 CAP	23 PIS	23 ARI
24 AQU	25 ARI	27 TAU	25 GEM	26 LEO	25 VIR	25 LIB	25 CAP	24 AQU	24 AQU	26 ARI	25 TAU
27 PIS	27 TAU	29 GEM	27 V1R	27 LIB	27 SCO	28 CAP	27 AQU	27 PIS	27 PIS	28 TAU	27 GEM
29 ARI	28 TAU	31 CAN	29 LEO	31 LIB	30 SCO	29 SAG	30 PIS	29 ARI	29 ARI	30 GEM	29 CAN
31 TAU			30 LEO			31 SAG			31 TAU		31 LEO

1956

JAN	FEB	MAR	APR	MAY	JUN	JUL	AUG	SEP	OCT	NOV	DEC
1 LEO	1 LIB	1 SCO	1 SAG	1 CAP	1 PIS	1 ARI	1 TAU	1 CAN	1 LEO	1 LIB	1 SCO
2 VIR	3 SCO	4 SAG	3 CAP	3 AQU	3 ARI	3 TAU	2 GEM	2 LEO	2 VIR	2 SCO	2 SAG
4 LIB	6 SAG	6 CAP	5 AQU	5 PIS	6 TAU	6 GEM	4 CAN	4 VIR	4 LIB	5 SAG	4 CAP
7 SCO	8 CAP	9 AQU	7 PIS	7 ARI	8 GEM	8 CAN	6 LEO	7 LIB	6 SCO	7 CAP	7 AQU
9 SAG	11 AQU	11 PIS	10 ARI	10 TAU	10 CAN	10 LEO	8 VIR	9 SCO	8 SAG	10 AQU	9 PIS
12 CAP	13 PIS	14 ARI	12 TAU	12 GEM	12 LEO	12 VIR	10 LIB	12 SAG	11 CAP	12 PIS	12 ARI
14 AQU	15 ARI	16 TAU	14 GEM	14 CAN	14 VIR	14 LIB	12 SCO	15 CAP	13 AQU	15 ARI	14 TAU
17 PIS	18 TAU	18 GEM	17 CAN	16 LEO	16 LIB	16 SCO	15 SAG	16 AQU	16 PIS	17 TAU	17 GEM
19 ARI	20 GEM	20 CAN	19 LEO	18 VIR	19 SCO	18 SAG	17 CAP	18 PIS	18 ARI	19 GEM	19 CAN
21 TAU	22 CAN	22 LEO	21 VIR	20 LIB	21 SAG	21 CAP	20 AQU	22 PIS	21 TAU	21 CAN	21 LEO
24 GEM	24 LEO	24 VIR	23 LIB	22 SCO	24 CAP	23 AQU	22 PIS	23 TAU	23 GEM	23 LEO	23 VIR
26 CAN	26 VIR	27 LIB	25 SCO	25 SAG	26 AQU	26 PIS	25 ARI	25 GEM	25 CAN	25 VIR	25 LIB
28 LEO	28 LIB	29 SCO	28 SAG	27 CAP	29 PIS	28 ARI	27 TAU	27 CAN	27 LEO	28 LIB	27 SCO
30 VIR	29 LIB	31 SAG	30 CAP	30 AQU	30 PIS	31 TAU	29 GEM	29 LEO	29 VIR	30 SCO	29 SAG
31 VIR				31 AQU			31 CAN		31 LIB		31 SAG

1957

JAN	FEB	MAR	APR	MAY	JUN	JUL	AUG	SEP	OCT	NOV	DEC
1 CAP	1 AQU	1 PIS	1 ARI	1 TAU	1 CAN	1 LEO	1 LIB	1 SAG	1 CAP	1 AQU	1 PIS
3 AQU	2 PIS	4 ARI	2 TAU	2 GEM	3 LEO	2 VIR	3 SCO	3 CAP	3 AQU	2 PIS	2 ARI
6 PIS	5 ARI	6 TAU	5 GEM	4 CAN	5 VIR	4 LIB	5 SAG	6 AQU	6 PIS	4 ARI	4 TAU
8 ARI	7 TAU	9 GEM	7 CAN	6 LEO	7 LIB	6 SCO	7 CAP	8 PIS	8 ARI	7 TAU	7 GEM
11 TAU	9 GEM	11 CAN	9 LEO	9 VIR	9 SCO	9 SAG	10 AQU	11 ARI	11 TAU	9 GEM	9 CAN
13 GEM	11 CAN	13 LEO	11 VIR	11 LIB	11 SAG	11 CAP	12 PIS	13 TAU	13 GEM	12 CAN	11 LEO
15 CAN	14 LEO	15 VIR	13 LIB	13 SCO	14 CAP	13 AQU	15 ARI	16 GEM	15 CAN	14 LEO	13 VIR
17 LEO	15 VIR	17 LIB	15 SCO	15 SAG	16 AQU	16 PIS	17 TAU	18 CAN	18 LEO	16 VIR	15 LIB
19 VIR	17 LIB	19 SCO	18 SAG	17 CAP	19 PIS	18 ARI	20 GEM	20 LEO	20 VIR	18 LIB	17 SCO
21 LIB	20 SCO	21 SAG	20 CAP	20 AQU	21 ARI	21 TAU	22 CAN	22 VIR	22 LIB	20 SCO	20 SAG
23 SCO	22 SAG	24 CAP	22 AQU	22 PIS	23 TAU	23 GEM	24 LEO	24 LIB	24 SCO	22 SAG	22 CAP
26 SAG	24 CAP	26 ACU	25 PIS	25 ARI	26 GEM	25 CAN	25 VIR	26 SCO	26 SAG	24 CAP	24 AQU
28 CAP	27 AQU	29 PIS	27 ARI	27 TAU	28 CAN	27 LEO	28 LIB	28 SAG	28 CAP	27 AQU	27 PIS
30 AQU	28 ACU	31 ARI	30 TAU	29 GEM	30 LEO	29 VIR	30 SCO	30 SAG	30 AQU	29 PIS	29 ARI
31 AQU				31 GEM		31 LIB	31 SCO		31 AQU	30 PIS	31 ARI

242

Moon Ephemeris: How to Find Your Moon Sign

1958

JAN	FEB	MAR	APR	MAY	JUN	JUL	AUG	SEP	OCT	NOV	DEC
1 TAU	1 GEM	1 CAN	1 LEO	1 LIB	1 SCO	1 CAP	1 AQU	1 ARI	1 TAU	1 GEM	1 LEO
3 GEM	2 CAN	3 LEO	2 VIR	3 SCO	2 SAG	3 AQU	2 PIS	3 TAU	3 GEM	2 CAN	4 VIR
5 CAN	4 LEO	5 VIR	4 LIB	5 SAG	4 CAP	6 PIS	4 ARI	6 GEM	6 CAN	4 LEO	6 LIB
7 LEO	6 VIR	7 LIB	6 SCO	7 CAP	6 AQU	8 ARI	7 TAU	8 CAN	8 LEO	6 VIR	8 SCO
9 VIR	8 LIB	9 SCO	8 SAG	10 AQU	8 PIS	11 TAU	10 GEM	11 LEO	10 VIR	9 LIB	10 SAG
12 LIB	10 SCO	11 SAG	10 CAP	12 PIS	11 ARI	13 GEM	12 CAN	13 VIR	12 LIB	11 SCO	12 CAP
14 SCO	12 SAG	14 CAP	12 AQU	14 ARI	13 TAU	16 CAN	14 LEO	15 LIB	14 SCO	13 SAG	14 AQU
16 SAG	14 CAP	16 AQU	15 PIS	17 TAU	16 GEM	18 LEO	16 VIR	17 SCO	16 SAG	15 CAP	16 PIS
18 CAP	17 AQU	18 PIS	17 ARI	20 GEM	18 CAN	20 VIR	18 LIB	19 SAG	18 CAP	17 AQU	19 ARI
20 AQU	19 PIS	21 ARI	20 TAU	22 CAN	20 LEO	22 LIB	20 SCO	21 CAP	20 AQU	19 PIS	21 TAU
23 PIS	22 ARI	24 TAU	22 GEM	24 LEO	23 VIR	24 SCO	22 SAG	23 AQU	23 PIS	22 ARI	24 GEM
25 ARI	24 TAU	26 GEM	25 CAN	26 VIR	25 LIB	26 SAG	25 CAP	25 PIS	25 ARI	24 TAU	26 CAN
28 TAU	27 GEM	28 CAN	27 LEO	28 LIB	27 SCO	28 CAP	27 AQU	28 ARI	28 TAU	27 GEM	29 LEO
30 GEM	28 GEM	31 LEO	29 VIR	31 SCO	29 SAG	31 AQU	29 PIS	30 TAU	30 GEM	29 CAN	31 VIR
31 GEM			30 VIR		30 SAG		31 PIS		31 GEM	30 CAN	

1959

JAN	FEB	MAR	APR	MAY	JUN	JUL	AUG	SEP	OCT	NOV	DEC
1 VIR	1 SCO	1 SCO	1 CAP	1 AQU	1 ARI	1 TAU	1 GEM	1 LEO	1 VIR	1 SCO	1 SAG
2 LIB	3 SAG	2 SAG	2 AQU	2 PIS	3 TAU	3 GEM	2 CAN	3 VIR	2 LIB	3 SAG	2 CAP
4 SCO	5 CAP	4 CAP	5 PIS	4 ARI	6 GEM	6 CAN	4 LEO	5 LIB	4 SCO	5 CAP	4 AQU
6 SAG	7 AQU	6 AQU	7 ARI	7 TAU	8 CAN	8 LEO	7 VIR	7 SCO	7 SAG	7 AQU	7 PIS
8 CAP	9 PIS	9 PIS	10 TAU	9 GEM	11 LEO	10 VIR	9 LIB	9 SAG	9 CAP	9 PIS	9 ARI
11 AQU	12 ARI	11 ARI	12 GEM	12 CAN	13 VIR	13 LIB	11 SCO	11 CAP	11 AQU	12 ARI	11 TAU
13 PIS	14 TAU	13 TAU	15 CAN	14 LEO	15 LIB	15 SCO	13 SAG	14 AQU	13 PIS	14 TAU	14 GEM
15 ARI	17 GEM	16 GEM	17 LEO	17 VIR	17 SCO	17 SAG	15 CAP	16 PIS	15 ARI	17 GEM	16 CAN
18 TAU	19 CAN	18 CAN	19 VIR	19 LIB	19 SAG	19 CAP	17 AQU	18 ARI	18 TAU	19 CAN	19 LEO
20 GEM	21 LEO	21 LEO	22 LIB	21 SCO	21 CAP	21 AQU	19 PIS	20 TAU	20 GEM	22 LEO	21 VIR
23 CAN	24 VIR	23 VIR	24 SCO	23 SAG	23 AQU	23 PIS	22 ARI	23 GEM	23 CAN	24 VIR	24 LIB
25 LEO	26 LIB	25 LIB	26 SAG	25 CAP	26 P15	25 ARI	24 TAU	25 CAN	25 LEO	26 LIB	26 SCO
27 VIR	28 SCO	27 SCO	28 CAP	27 AQU	28 ARI	28 TAU	27 GEM	28 LEO	28 VIR	28 SCO	28 SAG
29 LIB		29 SAG	30 AQU	29 PIS	30 TAU	30 GEM	29 CAN	30 VIR	30 LIB	30 SAG	30 CAP
31 LIB		31 CAP		31 PIS			31 GEM		31 LIB		31 CAP

1960

JAN	FEB	MAR	APR	MAY	JUN	JUL	AUG	SEP	OCT	NOV	DEC
1 AQU	1 PIS	1 ARI	1 GEM	1 CAN	1 LEO	1 VIR	1 SCO	1 CAP	1 AQU	1 ARI	1 TAU
3 PIS	2 ARI	2 TAU	4 CAN	3 LEO	2 VIR	2 LIB	3 SAG	3 AQU	2 PIS	3 TAU	3 GEM
5 ARI	4 TAU	5 GEM	6 LEO	6 VIR	4 SCO	5 CAP	5 PIS	5 ARI	5 TAU	5 GEM	5 CAN
8 TAU	6 GEM	7 CAN	9 VIR	8 LIB	7 SCO	6 SAG	7 AQU	7 ARI	7 GEM	8 CAN	8 LEO
10 GEM	9 CAN	10 LEO	11 LIB	10 SCO	9 SAG	9 CAP	9 PIS	9 TAU	9 GEM	10 LEO	10 VIR
13 CAN	11 LEO	12 VIR	13 SCO	12 SAG	11 CAP	10 AQU	11 ARI	12 GEM	12 CAN	13 VIR	13 LIB
15 LEO	14 VIR	14 LIB	15 SAG	14 CAP	14 AQU	12 PIS	13 TAU	14 CAN	14 LEO	15 LIB	15 SCO
18 VIR	16 LIB	17 SCO	17 CAP	17 AQU	15 GEM	14 ARI	15 GEM	17 LEO	17 VIR	17 SCO	17 SAG
20 LIB	18 SCO	19 SAG	19 AQU	19 PIS	17 ARI	17 TAU	18 CAN	19 VIR	19 LIB	19 SAG	19 CAP
22 SCO	20 SAG	21 CAP	21 PIS	21 ARI	19 TAU	19 GEM	20 LEO	22 LIB	21 SCO	22 CAP	21 AQU
24 SAG	23 CAP	23 AQU	23 ARI	23 TAU	22 GEM	22 CAN	23 VIR	24 SCO	23 SAG	24 AQU	23 PIS
26 CAP	25 AQU	25 PIS	26 TAU	26 GEM	24 CAN	24 LEO	25 LIB	26 SAG	25 CAP	26 PIS	25 ARI
28 AQU	27 PIS	27 ARI	28 GEM	28 CAN	27 LEO	27 VIR	28 SCO	28 CAP	28 AQU	28 ARI	28 TAU
30 PIS	29 ARI	30 TAU	30 CAN	31 LEO	29 VIR	29 LIB	30 SAG	30 AQU	30 PIS	30 TAU	30 GEM
31 PIS		31 TAU				31 SCO	31 SAG				31 GEM

1961

JAN	FEB	MAR	APR	MAY	JUN	JUL	AUG	SEP	OCT	NOV	DEC
1 GEM	1 LEO	1 LEO	1 LIB	1 SCO	1 CAP	1 AQU	1 AQI	1 TAU	1 CAN	1 LEO	1 VIR
2 CAN	3 VIR	2 VIR	3 SCO	3 SAG	3 AQU	3 P15	3 TAU	2 GEM	4 LEO	3 VIR	3 LIB
4 LEO	5 LIB	5 LIB	5 SAG	5 CAP	5 PIS	5 ARI	5 GEM	4 CAN	6 VIR	5 LIB	5 SCO
7 VIR	8 SCO	7 SCO	8 CAP	7 AQU	7 ARI	7 TAU	8 CAN	7 LEO	9 LIB	8 SCO	7 SAG
9 LIB	10 SAG	9 SAG	10 AQU	9 PIS	10 TAU	9 GEM	10 LEO	9 VIR	11 SCO	10 SAG	10 CAP
11 SCO	12 CAP	11 CAP	12 PIS	11 ARI	12 GEM	12 CAN	13 VIR	12 LIB	13 SAG	12 CAP	12 AQU
14 SAG	14 AQU	13 AQU	14 ARI	13 TAU	14 CAN	14 LEO	15 LIB	14 SCO	15 CAP	14 AQU	14 PIS
16 CAP	16 PIS	16 PIS	16 TAU	16 GEM	17 LEO	17 VIR	18 SCO	16 SAG	18 AQU	17 PIS	16 ARI
18 AQU	18 ARI	18 ARI	18 GEM	18 CAN	19 VIR	19 LIB	20 SAG	19 CAP	20 PIS	19 ARI	18 TAU
20 PIS	20 TAU	20 TAU	21 CAN	21 LEO	22 LIB	22 SCO	22 CAP	21 AQU	22 ARI	21 TAU	20 GEM
22 ARI	23 GEM	22 GEM	23 LEO	23 VIR	24 SCO	24 SAG	24 AQU	23 PIS	24 TAU	23 GEM	23 CAN
24 TAU	25 CAN	24 CAN	26 VIR	26 LIB	26 SAG	26 CAP	26 PIS	25 ARI	27 GEM	25 CAN	25 LEO
26 GEM	28 LEO	27 LEO	28 LIB	28 SCO	29 CAP	29 AQU	28 ARI	27 TAU	29 CAN	28 LEO	27 VIR
29 CAN		29 VIR	30 LIB	30 SAG	30 CAP	31 PIS	31 TAU	29 GEM	30 GEM	30 LIB	30 LIB
31 LEO		31 VIR		31 SAG				30 GEM			31 LIB

1962

JAN	FEB	MAR	APR	MAY	JUN	JUL	AUG	SEP	OCT	NOV	DEC
1 SCO	1 SAG	1 SAG	1 AQU	1 PIS	1 TAU	1 GEM	1 LEO	1 VIR	1 SCO	1 SAG	1 CAP
4 SAG	2 CAP	2 CAP	2 PIS	2 AQU	2 GEM	2 CAN	3 VIR	2 LIB	4 SAG	3 CAP	2 AQU
6 CAP	4 AQU	4 AQU	4 ARI	4 TAU	4 CAN	5 LEO	5 LIB	4 SCO	6 CAP	5 AQU	4 PIS
8 AQU	6 PIS	6 PIS	6 TAU	6 GEM	7 LEO	7 VIR	8 SCO	7 SAG	9 AQU	7 PIS	6 ARI
10 PIS	8 ARI	8 ARI	8 GEM	8 CAN	9 VIR	9 LIB	10 SAG	9 CAP	11 PIS	9 ARI	9 TAU
12 ARI	11 TAU	10 TAU	11 CAN	11 LEO	12 LIB	12 SCO	13 CAP	11 AQU	13 ARI	11 TAU	11 GEM
14 TAU	12 GEM	12 GEM	13 LEO	13 VIR	14 SCO	14 SAG	15 AQU	13 PIS	15 TAU	13 GEM	13 CAN
16 GEM	15 CAN	14 CAN	16 VIQ	15 LIB	17 SAG	16 CAP	17 PIS	15 ARI	17 GEM	15 CAN	15 LEO
19 CAN	18 LEO	17 LEO	18 LIB	18 SCO	20 PIS	18 AQU	19 ARI	17 TAU	19 CAN	17 LEO	17 VIR
21 LEO	20 VIR	19 VIR	21 SCO	20 SAG	22 PIS	21 PIS	21 TAU	19 GEM	21 LEO	19 VIR	20 LIB
24 VIR	23 LIB	21 LIB	23 SAG	22 CAP	23 ARI	22 GEM	23 CAN	22 LEO	24 VIR	22 LIB	22 SCO
26 LIB	25 SCO	24 SCO	25 CAP	25 AQU	25 TAU	24 LEO	24 LEO	26 LIB	26 LIB	25 SCO	25 SAG
29 SCO	27 SAG	26 SAG	28 AQU	27 PIS	27 GEM	28 LEO	26 VIR	29 SCO	29 SAG	25 SCO	27 CAP
31 SAG	28 SAG	29 CAP	30 PIS	29 ARI	30 GEM	30 VIR	29 LIB	31 SAG	31 SCO	27 CAP	29 AQU
		31 AQU		31 TAU			31 LEO		31 VIR	30 LIB	31 AQU

~ *Healing Mind, Body, Spirit*

1963

JAN	FEB	MAR	APR	MAY	JUN	JUL	AUG	SEP	OCT	NOV	DEC
1 PIS	1 TAU	1 TAU	1 CAN	1 LEO	1 VIR	1 SCO	1 SAG	1 AQU	1 PIS	1 ARI	1 GEM
2 ARI	3 GEM	2 GEM	3 LEO	3 VIR	2 LIB	4 SAG	3 CAP	4 PIS	2 ARI	2 TAU	3 CAN
5 TAU	5 CAN	5 CAN	6 VIR	5 LIB	4 SCO	6 CAP	5 AQU	6 ARI	5 TAU	3 GEM	5 LEO
7 GEM	8 LEO	7 LEO	8 LIB	8 SCO	7 SAG	9 AQU	7 PIS	8 TAU	7 GEM	6 CAN	7 VIR
9 CAN	10 VIR	9 VIR	11 SCO	10 SAG	9 CAP	11 PIS	9 ARI	10 GEM	9 CAN	8 LEO	10 LIB
11 LEO	12 LIB	11 LIB	13 SAG	13 CAP	11 AQU	13 ARI	11 TAU	12 CAN	11 LEO	10 VIR	12 SCO
14 VIR	15 SCO	14 SCO	16 CAP	15 AQU	14 PIS	15 TAU	14 GEM	14 LEO	14 VIR	12 LIB	15 SAG
16 LIB	17 SAG	17 SAG	18 AQU	17 PIS	16 ARI	17 GEM	16 CAN	16 VIR	16 LIB	15 SCO	17 CAP
19 SCO	20 CAP	19 CAP	20 PIS	20 ARI	18 TAU	19 CAN	18 LEO	19 LIB	19 SCO	17 SAG	20 AQU
21 SAG	22 AQU	22 AQU	22 ARI	22 TAU	20 GEM	22 LEO	21 SCO	21 SCO	22 CAP	22 AQU	22 PIS
23 CAP	24 PIS	24 PIS	24 TAU	24 GEM	22 CAN	24 VIR	23 LIB	24 SAG	24 CAP	22 AQU	24 ARI
26 AQU	26 ARI	26 ARI	26 GEM	26 CAN	24 LEO	26 LIB	25 SCO	26 CAP	26 AQU	25 PIS	26 TAU
28 PIS	28 TAU	28 TAU	28 CAN	28 LEO	26 VIR	29 SCO	28 SAG	29 AQU	28 PIS	27 ARI	28 GEM
30 ARI		30 GEM	30 LEO	30 VIR	29 LIB	31 SAG	30 CAP	30 AQU	31 ARI	29 TAU	30 CAN
31 ARI		31 GEM		31 VIR	30 LIB					30 TAU	31 CAN

1964

JAN	FEB	MAR	APR	MAY	JUN	JUL	AUG	SEP	OCT	NOV	DEC
1 LEO	1 VIR	1 LIB	1 SCO	1 SAG	1 AQU	1 PIS	1 TAU	1 GEM	1 LEO	1 VIR	1 SCO
4 VIR	2 LIB	3 SCO	2 SAG	2 CAP	3 PIS	3 ARI	3 GEM	2 CAN	3 VIR	2 LIB	4 SAG
6 LIB	5 SCO	6 SAG	4 CAP	4 AQU	5 ARI	5 TAU	5 CAN	4 LEO	5 LIB	4 SCO	6 CAP
8 SCO	7 SAG	8 CAP	7 AQU	7 PIS	7 TAU	7 GEM	7 LEO	6 VIR	8 SCO	6 SAG	9 AQU
11 SAG	10 CAP	11 AQU	9 PIS	9 ARI	9 GEM	9 CAN	9 VIR	8 LIB	10 SAG	9 CAP	11 PIS
13 CAP	12 AQU	13 PIS	11 ARI	11 TAU	11 CAN	11 LEO	11 LIB	10 SCO	12 CAP	11 AQU	14 ARI
16 AQU	15 PIS	15 ARI	14 TAU	13 GEM	13 LEO	13 VIR	14 SCO	13 SAG	15 AQU	14 PIS	16 TAU
13 PIS	17 ARI	17 TAU	16 GEM	15 CAN	15 VIR	15 LIB	16 SAG	15 CAP	17 PIS	16 ARI	18 GEM
20 ARI	19 TAU	19 GEM	18 CAN	17 LEO	18 LIB	17 SCO	19 CAP	18 AQU	20 ARI	18 TAU	20 CAN
23 TAU	21 GEM	21 CAN	20 LEO	19 VIR	20 SCO	20 SAG	21 AQU	20 PIS	22 TAU	20 GEM	22 LEO
25 GEM	23 CAN	24 LEO	22 VIR	22 LIB	23 SAG	23 CAP	24 PIS	22 ARI	24 GEM	22 CAN	24 VIR
27 CAN	25 LEO	26 VIR	24 LIB	24 SCO	25 CAP	25 AQU	26 ARI	24 TAU	26 CAN	24 LEO	26 LIB
29 LEO	27 VIR	28 LIB	27 SCO	26 SAG	28 AQU	27 PIS	28 TAU	27 GEM	28 LEO	27 VIR	28 SCO
31 VIR	29 VIR	30 SCO	29 SAG	29 CAP	30 PIS	30 ARI	30 GEM	29 CAN	30 VIR	29 LIB	31 SAG
		31 SCO	30 SAG	31 CAP			31 ARI	31 GEM	30 CAN	31 VIR	30 LIB

1965

JAN	FEB	MAR	APR	MAY	JUN	JUL	AUG	SEP	OCT	NOV	DEC
1 SAG	1 AQU	1 AQU	1 PIS	1 TAU	1 GEM	1 LEO	1 VIR	1 LEO	1 SAG	1 AQU	1 PIS
2 CAP	4 PIS	3 PIS	2 ARI	3 GEM	2 CAN	3 VIR	2 LIB	2 SAG	2 CAP	4 PIS	3 ARI
5 AQU	6 ARI	5 ARI	4 TAU	5 CAN	4 LEO	5 LIB	4 SCO	5 CAP	5 AQU	6 ARI	6 TAU
7 PIS	8 TAU	8 TAU	6 GEM	8 LEO	6 VIR	8 SCO	6 SAG	7 AQU	7 PIS	8 TAU	8 GEM
10 ARI	11 GEM	10 GEM	8 CAN	10 VIR	8 LIB	10 SAG	9 CAP	9 PIS	10 ARI	11 GEM	10 CAN
12 TAU	13 CAN	12 CAN	10 LEO	12 LIB	10 SCO	12 CAP	11 AQU	12 ARI	12 TAU	13 CAN	12 LEO
14 GEM	15 LEO	14 LEO	12 VIR	14 SCO	13 SAG	15 AQU	14 PIS	14 TAU	14 GEM	15 LEO	14 VIR
16 CAN	17 VIR	16 VIR	15 LIB	16 SAG	15 CAP	17 PIS	16 ARI	17 GEM	17 CAN	17 VIR	16 LIB
18 LEO	19 LIB	18 LIB	17 SCO	19 CAP	18 AQU	20 ARI	19 TAU	19 CAN	19 LEO	19 LIB	19 SCO
20 VIR	21 SCO	20 SCO	19 SAG	21 AQU	20 PIS	22 TAU	21 GEM	21 LEO	21 VIR	21 SCO	21 SAG
22 LIB	23 SAG	23 SAG	22 CAP	24 PIS	23 ARI	25 GEM	23 CAN	23 VIR	23 LIB	24 SAG	23 CAP
25 SCO	26 CAP	25 CAP	24 AQU	26 ARI	25 TAU	27 CAN	25 LEO	26 LIB	25 SCO	26 CAP	26 AQU
27 SAG	28 AQU	28 AQU	27 PIS	29 TAU	27 GEM	29 LEO	27 VIR	28 SCO	27 SAG	28 AQU	28 PIS
30 CAP		30 PIS	29 ARI	31 GEM	29 CAN	31 VIR	29 LIB	30 SAG	30 CAP	30 AQU	31 ARI
31 CAP		31 PIS	30 ARI		30 CAN		31 SCO		31 CAP		

1966

JAN	FEB	MAR	APR	MAY	JUN	JUL	AUG	SEP	OCT	NOV	DEC
1 ARI	1 GEM	1 GEM	1 LEO	1 VIR	1 SCO	1 SAG	1 AQU	1 PIS	1 ARI	1 GEM	1 CAN
2 TAU	3 CAN	2 CAN	3 VIR	2 LIB	3 SAG	2 CAP	4 PIS	2 ARI	2 TAU	3 CAN	3 LEO
5 GEM	5 LEO	5 LEO	5 LIB	4 SCO	5 CAP	5 AQU	6 ARI	5 GEM	5 CAN	5 LEO	5 VIR
7 CAN	7 VIR	7 VIR	7 SCO	7 SAG	8 AQU	7 PIS	9 TAU	7 CAN	7 LEO	8 VIR	7 LIB
9 LEO	9 LIB	9 LIB	9 SAG	9 CAP	10 PIS	10 ARI	11 GEM	9 LEO	9 VIR	10 LIB	9 SCO
11 VIR	11 SCO	11 SCO	11 CAP	11 AQU	13 ARI	12 TAU	13 CAN	12 LEO	11 VIR	12 SCO	11 SAG
13 LIB	13 SAG	13 SAG	14 AQU	14 PIS	15 TAU	15 GEM	15 LEO	14 VIR	13 LIB	14 SAG	14 CAP
15 SCO	16 CAP	15 CAP	16 PIS	16 ARI	17 GEM	17 CAN	17 VIR	16 LIB	15 SCO	16 CAP	16 AQU
17 SAG	18 AQU	18 AQU	19 ARI	19 TAU	20 CAN	19 LEO	19 LIB	18 SCO	17 SAG	18 AQU	18 PIS
20 CAP	21 PIS	20 PIS	21 TAU	21 GEM	22 LEO	21 VIR	21 SCO	20 SAG	20 CAP	21 PIS	21 ARI
22 AQU	23 ARI	23 ARI	24 GEM	23 CAN	24 VIR	23 LIB	24 SAG	22 CAP	22 AQU	23 ARI	23 TAU
25 PIS	26 TAU	25 TAU	26 CAN	25 LEO	26 LIB	25 SCO	26 CAP	25 AQU	24 PIS	26 TAU	26 CAN
27 ARI	28 GEM	27 GEM	28 LEO	27 VIR	28 SCO	27 SAG	28 AQU	27 PIS	27 ARI	28 GEM	28 CAN
30 TAU		30 CAN	30 VIR	30 LIB	30 SCO	30 CAP	31 PIS	30 ARI	29 TAU	30 CAN	30 LEO
31 TAU		31 CAN		31 LIB		31 CAP			31 TAU		31 LEO

1967

JAN	FEB	MAR	APR	MAY	JUN	JUL	AUG	SEP	OCT	NOV	DEC
1 VIR	1 LIB	1 SCO	1 SAG	1 AQU	1 PIS	1 ARI	1 GEM	1 CAN	1 LEO	1 LIB	1 SCO
3 LIB	2 SCO	3 SAG	2 CAP	4 PIS	2 ARI	2 TAU	3 CAN	2 LEO	2 VIR	2 SCO	2 SAG
5 SCO	4 SAG	5 CAP	4 AQU	6 ARI	5 TAU	5 GEM	6 LEO	4 VIR	4 LIB	4 SAG	4 CAP
8 SAG	6 CAP	8 AQU	6 PIS	9 TAU	7 GEM	7 CAN	8 VIR	6 LIB	6 SCO	6 CAP	6 AQU
10 CAP	8 AQU	10 PIS	9 ARI	11 GEM	10 CAN	12 LEO	10 LIB	8 SCO	8 SAG	8 AQU	8 PIS
12 AQU	11 PIS	13 ARI	11 TAU	14 CAN	12 LEO	12 VIR	12 SCO	10 SAG	10 CAP	11 PIS	10 ARI
14 PIS	13 ARI	15 TAU	14 GEM	16 LEO	14 VIR	14 LIB	14 SAG	12 CAP	12 AQU	13 ARI	13 TAU
17 ARI	16 TAU	18 GEM	16 CAN	18 VIR	16 LIB	16 SCO	16 CAP	15 AQU	14 PIS	17 ARI	15 GEM
19 TAU	18 GEM	20 CAN	20 LIB	20 LIB	19 SAG	18 SAG	19 AQU	17 PIS	17 ARI	18 GEM	18 CAN
22 GEM	21 CAN	22 LEO	21 VIR	22 SCO	21 SAG	20 CAP	22 PIS	19 ARI	19 TAU	21 CAN	20 LEO
24 CAN	23 LEO	24 VIR	23 LIB	24 SAG	23 CAP	22 AQU	23 ARI	22 TAU	22 GEM	23 LEO	23 VIR
26 LEO	25 VIR	26 LIB	25 SCO	26 CAP	25 AQU	25 PIS	25 TAU	25 GEM	24 CAN	25 VIR	25 LIB
28 VIR	27 LIB	28 SCO	27 SAG	28 AQU	27 PIS	27 ARI	27 GEM	27 CAN	27 LEO	28 LIB	27 SCO
30 LIB	28 LIB	30 SAG	29 CAP	31 PIS	30 ARI	30 TAU	31 CAN	30 LEO	29 VIR	30 SCO	29 SAG
31 LIB		31 SAG	30 CAP			31 TAU			31 LIB		31 CAP

244

Moon Ephemeris: How to Find Your Moon Sign

1968

JAN	FEB	MAR	APR	MAY	JUN	JUL	AUG	SEP	OCT	NOV	DEC
1 CAP	1 PIS	1 ARI	1 TAU	1 GEM	1 LEO	1 VIR	1 LIB	1 SAG	1 AQU	1 PIS	1 ARI
2 AQU	3 ARI	4 TAU	3 GEM	3 CAN	4 VIR	3 LIB	2 SCO	2 CAP	4 PIS	2 ARI	2 TAU
4 PIS	6 TAU	6 GEM	5 CAN	5 LEO	6 LIB	5 SCO	4 SAG	4 AQU	6 ARI	5 TAU	4 GEM
7 ARI	8 GEM	9 CAN	8 LEO	7 VIR	8 SCO	7 SAG	6 CAP	6 PIS	8 TAU	7 GEM	7 CAN
9 TAU	11 CAN	11 LEO	10 VIR	10 LIB	10 SAG	9 CAP	8 AQU	9 ARI	11 GEM	10 CAN	9 LEO
12 GEM	13 LEO	14 VIR	12 LIB	12 SCO	12 CAP	11 AQU	10 PIS	11 TAU	13 CAN	12 LEO	12 VIR
14 CAN	15 VIR	16 LIB	14 SCO	14 SAG	14 AQU	14 PIS	12 ARI	13 GEM	16 LEO	15 VIR	14 LIB
17 LEO	17 LIB	18 SCO	16 SAG	16 CAP	16 PIS	15 TAU	15 TAU	16 CAN	18 VIR	17 LIB	16 SCO
19 VIR	19 SCO	20 SAG	18 SCO	18 AQU	19 ARI	18 TAU	17 GEM	18 LEO	20 LIB	19 SCO	18 SAG
21 LIB	22 SAG	22 CAP	20 AQU	20 PIS	21 TAU	20 GEM	20 CAN	21 VIR	23 SCO	21 SAG	20 CAP
23 SCO	24 CAP	24 AQU	23 PIS	22 ARI	24 GEM	23 CAN	22 LEO	23 LIB	25 SAG	23 CAP	22 AQU
25 SAG	26 AQU	26 PIS	25 ARI	25 TAU	26 CAN	25 LEO	25 VIR	25 SCO	27 CAP	25 AQU	24 PIS
27 CAP	28 PIS	29 ARI	28 TAU	27 GEM	29 LEO	28 VIR	27 LIB	27 SAG	29 AQU	27 PIS	27 ARI
30 AQU	29 PIS	31 TAU	30 GEM	30 CAN	30 LEO	30 LIB	29 SCO	29 CAP	31 PIS	29 ARI	29 TAU
31 AQU				31 CAN			31 LIB			30 ARI	31 TAU

1969

JAN	FEB	MAR	APR	MAY	JUN	JUL	AUG	SEP	OCT	NOV	DEC
1 GEM	1 CAN	1 LEO	1 VIR	1 VIR	1 SAG	1 SAG	1 PIS	1 TAU	1 GEM	1 CAN	1 LEO
3 CAN	2 LEO	4 VIR	2 LIB	2 SCO	2 CAP	2 AQU	2 ARI	3 GEM	3 CAN	2 LEO	2 VIR
6 LEO	4 VIR	6 LIB	5 SCO	4 SAG	4 AQU	4 PIS	4 TAU	6 CAN	6 LEO	5 VIR	4 LIB
8 VIR	7 LIB	8 SCO	7 SAG	6 CAP	6 PIS	6 ARI	6 GEM	8 LEO	8 VIR	7 LIB	7 SCO
10 LIB	9 SCO	10 SAG	9 CAP	8 AQU	9 ARI	9 TAU	9 CAN	11 VIR	11 LIB	9 SCO	9 SAG
13 SCO	11 SAG	12 CAP	11 AQU	10 PIS	11 TAU	11 GEM	12 LEO	13 LIB	13 SCO	11 SAG	11 CAP
15 SAG	13 CAP	15 AQU	13 PIS	12 ARI	13 GEM	13 CAN	15 VIR	16 SCO	15 SAG	13 CAP	13 AQU
17 CAP	15 AQU	17 PIS	15 ARI	15 TAU	16 CAN	16 LEO	17 LIB	18 SAG	17 CAP	15 AQU	15 PIS
19 AQU	17 PIS	19 ARI	18 TAU	17 GEM	19 LEO	18 VIR	19 SCO	20 CAP	19 AQU	18 PIS	17 ARI
21 PIS	19 ARI	21 TAU	20 GEM	20 CAN	21 VIR	21 LIB	22 SAG	22 AQU	21 PIS	20 ARI	19 TAU
23 ARI	22 TAU	24 GEM	22 CAN	22 LEO	23 LIB	23 SCO	24 CAP	24 PIS	24 ARI	22 TAU	22 GEM
25 TAU	24 GEM	26 CAN	25 LEO	25 VIR	26 SCO	25 SAG	26 AQU	26 ARI	26 TAU	24 GEM	24 CAN
28 GEM	27 CAN	29 LEO	27 VIR	27 LIB	28 SAG	27 CAP	28 PIS	28 TAU	28 GEM	27 CAN	27 LEO
30 CAN	28 CAN	31 VIR	30 LIB	29 SCO	30 CAP	29 AQU	30 ARI	30 TAU	30 CAN	29 LEO	29 VIR
31 CAN				31 SAG		31 PIS	31 ARI		31 CAN	30 LEO	31 VIR

1970

JAN	FEB	MAR	APR	MAY	JUN	JUL	AUG	SEP	OCT	NOV	DEC
1 LIB	1 SCO	1 SAG	1 AQU	1 PIS	1 TAU	1 GEM	1 CAN	1 VIR	1 LIB	1 SCO	1 CAP
3 SCO	2 SAG	3 CAP	4 PIS	3 ARI	4 GEM	3 CAN	2 LEO	3 LIB	3 SCO	2 SAG	3 AQU
5 SAG	4 CAP	5 AQU	6 ARI	5 TAU	6 CAN	6 LEO	4 VIR	6 SCO	5 SAG	4 CAP	5 PIS
7 CAP	6 AQU	7 PIS	8 TAU	7 GEM	8 LEO	8 VIR	6 LIB	8 SAG	8 CAP	6 AQU	8 ARI
9 AQU	8 PIS	9 ARI	10 TAU	10 CAN	11 VIR	11 LIB	9 SCO	10 CAP	10 AQU	8 PIS	10 TAU
11 PIS	10 ARI	11 TAU	12 CAN	12 LEO	13 LIB	13 SCO	12 SAG	12 AQU	12 PIS	10 ARI	12 GEM
13 ARI	12 TAU	13 GEM	15 LEO	15 VIR	16 SCO	15 SAG	15 CAP	14 PIS	15 ARI	13 TAU	14 CAN
16 TAU	14 GEM	16 CAN	17 VIR	17 LIB	18 SAG	18 CAP	16 AQU	16 ARI	16 TAU	14 GEM	16 LEO
18 GEM	17 CAN	18 LEO	20 LIB	19 SCO	20 CAP	20 AQU	18 PIS	18 TAU	19 GEM	19 LEO	19 VIR
20 CAN	19 LEO	21 VIR	22 SCO	22 SAG	22 AQU	22 PIS	20 ARI	21 GEM	20 CAN	19 LEO	22 LIB
23 LEO	22 VIR	23 LIB	24 SAG	24 CAP	24 PIS	24 ARI	22 TAU	23 CAN	23 LEO	22 VIR	24 SCO
25 VIR	24 LIB	26 SCO	27 CAP	26 AQU	26 ARI	26 TAU	24 GEM	25 LEO	25 VIR	24 LIB	26 SAG
28 LIB	27 SCO	28 SAG	29 AQU	28 PIS	29 TAU	28 GEM	27 CAN	28 VIR	28 LIB	27 SCO	29 CAP
30 SCO	28 SCO	30 CAP	31 AQU	30 ARI	31 ARI	30 CAN	29 LEO	30 VIR	30 SCO	29 SAG	31 AQU
31 SCO		31 CAP		31 ARI			31 CAN	31 LEO		30 SAG	

1971

JAN	FEB	MAR	APR	MAY	JUN	JUL	AUG	SEP	OCT	NOV	DEC
1 AQU	1 ARI	1 TAU	1 GEM	1 CAN	1 VIR	1 LIB	1 SCO	1 CAP	1 AQU	1 ARI	1 TAU
2 PIS	2 TAU	4 GEM	2 CAN	2 LEO	3 LIB	3 SCO	2 SAG	3 AQU	2 PIS	3 TAU	2 GEM
4 ARI	4 GEM	6 CAN	5 LEO	4 VIR	6 SCO	5 SAG	4 CAP	5 PIS	4 ARI	5 GEM	4 CAN
6 TAU	7 CAN	8 LEO	7 VIR	7 LIB	8 SAG	8 CAP	6 AQU	7 ARI	6 TAU	7 CAN	6 LEO
8 GEM	9 LEO	11 VIR	10 LIB	10 SCO	10 CAP	10 AQU	8 PIS	9 TAU	8 GEM	10 LEO	9 VIR
10 CAN	12 VIR	13 LIB	12 SCO	12 SAG	13 AQU	12 PIS	10 ARI	11 GEM	10 CAN	11 VIR	11 LIB
13 LEO	14 LIB	16 SCO	15 SAG	15 CAP	15 PIS	14 ARI	13 TAU	13 CAN	13 LEO	14 LIB	14 SCO
VIR	17 SCO	18 SAG	17 CAP	17 AQU	17 ARI	16 TAU	15 GEM	15 LEO	15 VIR	16 SCO	16 SAG
18 LIB	19 SAG	21 CAP	19 AQU	19 PIS	19 TAU	18 GEM	17 CAN	18 VIR	18 LIB	19 SAG	19 CAP
20 SCO	21 CAP	23 AQU	21 PIS	21 ARI	21 GEM	21 CAN	19 LEO	20 LIB	20 SCO	21 CAP	21 AQU
23 SAG	23 AQU	25 PIS	23 ARI	23 TAU	23 CAN	23 LEO	22 VIR	23 SCO	23 SAG	23 AQU	23 PIS
25 CAP	26 PIS	27 ARI	25 TAU	25 GEM	26 LEO	25 VIR	24 LIB	25 SAG	25 CAP	26 PIS	25 ARI
27 AQU	27 ARI	29 TAU	27 GEM	27 CAN	28 VIR	28 LIB	27 SCO	28 CAP	28 AQU	28 ARI	27 TAU
29 PIS	28 ARI	31 GEM	30 CAN	29 LEO	30 VIR	30 SCO	29 SAG	30 AQU	30 PIS	30 TAU	30 GEM
31 ARI				31 LEO		31 SCO	31 SAG		31 PIS		31 GEM

1972

JAN	FEB	MAR	APR	MAY	JUN	JUL	AUG	SEP	OCT	NOV	DEC
1 CAN	1 LEO	1 VIR	1 SCO	1 SAG	1 CAP	1 AQU	1 ARI	1 GEM	1 CAN	1 VIR	1 LIB
3 LEO	2 VIR	4 LIB	4 SAG	3 CAP	2 AQU	2 PIS	3 CAN	3 CAN	2 LEO	3 LIB	3 SCO
5 VIR	4 LIB	5 SCO	6 CAP	6 AQU	4 PIS	4 ARI	4 GEM	5 LEO	4 VIR	5 SCO	5 SAG
8 LIB	6 SCO	7 SAG	9 CAP	8 PIS	7 ARI	6 TAU	6 CAN	7 VIR	7 LIB	7 SAG	8 CAP
10 SCO	9 SAG	10 CAP	11 PIS	10 ARI	9 TAU	8 GEM	8 LEO	9 LIB	9 SCO	10 CAP	10 AQU
13 SAG	11 CAP	12 AQU	13 ARI	12 TAU	11 GEM	10 CAN	11 VIR	12 SCO	12 SAG	13 AQU	13 PIS
15 CAP	14 AQU	14 PIS	15 TAU	14 GEM	13 CAN	13 LEO	14 LIB	14 SAG	14 CAP	15 PIS	15 ARI
17 AQU	16 PIS	17 ARI	17 GEM	16 CAN	15 LEO	16 VIR	16 SCO	17 CAP	17 AQU	17 ARI	17 TAU
19 PIS	18 ARI	18 TAU	19 CAN	18 LEO	17 VIR	18 SAG	19 AQU	19 PIS	20 LIB	19 GEM	21 CAN
22 ARI	20 TAU	20 GEM	21 LEO	21 VIR	19 LIB	22 SCO	22 PIS	21 ARI	22 GEM	21 CAN	24 GEM
24 TAU	22 GEM	22 CAN	23 VIR	23 LIB	22 SCO	22 SAG	24 ARI	24 TAU	23 TAU	24 VIR	25 VIR
26 GEM	24 CAN	25 LEO	26 LIB	26 SCO	24 SAG	25 PIS	26 PIS	25 GEM	25 CAN	26 LEO	27 LIB
28 CAN	27 LEO	27 VIR	28 SCO	28 SAG	27 CAP	27 AQU	28 TAU	27 CAN	28 VIR	28 LIB	29 SCO
30 LEO	29 VIR	30 LIB	30 SCO	30 AQU	31 AQU	30 CAN	30 LEO	30 LIB	30 SAG	31 SCO	
31 LEO		31 LIB		30 AQU	31 ARI	31 GEM		31 LEO			31 SCO

245

Healing Mind, Body, Spirit

1973

JAN	FEB	MAR	APR	MAY	JUN	JUL	AUG	SEP	OCT	NOV	DEC
1 SAG	1 CAP	1 CAP	1 PIS	1 ARI	1 GEM	1 CAN	1 VIR	1 LIB	1 SAG	1 CAP	1 AQU
4 CAP	3 AQU	2 AQU	3 ARI	3 TAU	3 CAN	3 LIB	2 SCO	4 CAP	3 AQU	3 PIS
6 AQU	5 PIS	4 PIS	5 TAU	5 GEM	5 LEO	4 VIR	5 SCO	4 SAG	7 AQU	5 PIS	5 ARI
9 PIS	7 ARI	7 ARI	7 GEM	7 CAN	7 VIR	8 SAG	7 CAP	9 PIS	8 ARI	7 TAU
11 ARI	10 TAU	9 TAU	9 CAN	9 LEO	9 LIB	9 SCO	10 CAP	9 AQU	11 ARI	10 TAU	9 GEM
13 TAU	12 GEM	11 GEM	11 LEO	11 VIR	12 SCO	12 SAG	13 AQU	12 PIS	13 TAU	12 GEM	11 CAN
15 GEM	14 CAN	13 CAN	14 VIR	13 LIB	14 SAG	14 CAP	15 PIS	14 ARI	16 GEM	14 CAN	13 LEO
17 CAN	16 LEO	15 LEO	16 LIB	16 SCO	17 CAP	17 AQU	18 ARI	16 TAU	18 CAN	16 LEO	15 VIR
19 LEO	18 VIR	17 VIR	18 SCO	18 SAG	19 AQU	19 PIS	20 TAU	18 GEM	20 LEO	18 VIR	18 LIB
22 VIR	20 LIB	20 LIB	21 SAG	21 W	22 PIS	22 ARI	22 GEM	20 CAN	22 VIR	20 LIB	20 SCO
24 LIB	23 SCO	22 SCO	23 CAP	23 AQU	24 ARI	24 TAU	24 CAN	21 LEO	24 LIB	23 SCO	22 SAG
26 SCO	25 SAG	24 SAG	26 AQU	26 PIS	26 TAU	26 GEM	26 LEO	25 VIR	26 SCO	25 SAG	25 CAP
29 SAG	28 CAP	27 CAP	28 PIS	28 ARI	28 GEM	28 CAN	28 VIR	27 LIB	29 SAG	28 CAP	27 AQU
31 CAP		29 AQU	30 ARI	30 TAU	30 CAN	30 LEO	30 LIB	29 SCO	31 CAP	30 AQU	30 PIS
		31 AQU		31 TAU		31 LEO	30 SCO				31 PIS

1974

JAN	FEB	MAR	APR	MAY	JUN	JUL	AUG	SEP	OCT	NOV	DEC
1 ARI	1 TAU	1 GEM	1 CAN	1 VIR	1 LIB	1 CAP	1 CAP	1 AQU	1 ARI	1 TAU	1 GEM
4 TAU	2 GEM	4 CAN	2 LEO	3 LIB	3 SCO	2 SAG	3 AQU	2 PIS	4 TAU	2 GEM	2 CAN
6 GEM	4 CAN	6 LEO	4 VIR	6 SCO	5 SAG	4 CAP	5 PIS	4 ARI	6 GEM	4 CAN	4 LEO
8 CAN	6 LEO	8 VIR	6 LIB	8 SAG	7 CAP	7 AQU	8 ARI	6 TAU	8 CAN	7 LEO	6 VIR
10 LEO	8 VIR	10 LIB	8 SCO	10 CAP	9 AQU	9 PIS	10 TAU	9 GEM	10 LEO	9 VIR	8 LIB
12 VIR	10 LIB	12 SCO	11 SAG	13 AQU	12 PIS	12 ARI	12 GEM	11 CAN	12 VIR	11 LIB	10 SCO
14 LIB	13 SCO	14 SAG	13 CAP	15 PIS	14 ARI	14 TAU	15 CAN	13 LEO	15 LIB	13 SCO	13 SAG
16 SCO	15 SAG	17 CAP	16 AQU	18 ARI	17 TAU	16 GEM	17 LEO	15 VIR	17 SCO	15 SAG	15 CAP
19 SAG	17 CAP	19 AQU	18 PIS	20 TAU	19 GEM	18 CAN	19 VIR	17 LIB	19 SAG	18 CAP	17 AQU
21 CAP	20 AQU	22 PIS	21 ARI	22 GEM	21 CAN	20 LEO	21 LIB	19 SCO	21 CAP	20 AQU	20 PIS
24 AQU	22 PIS	24 ARI	23 TAU	24 CAN	23 LEO	22 VIR	23 SCO	21 SAG	24 AQU	23 PIS	22 ARI
26 PIS	25 ARI	26 TAU	25 GEM	26 LEO	25 VIR	24 LIB	25 SAG	24 CAP	26 PIS	25 ARI	25 TAU
29 ARI	27 TAU	29 GEM	27 CAN	29 VIR	27 LIB	26 SCO	28 CAP	26 AQU	29 ARI	27 TAU	27 GEM
31 TAU	28 TAU	31 CAN	29 LEO	31 LIB	29 SCO	29 SAG	30 AQU	29 PIS	31 TAU	30 GEM	29 CAN
			30 LEO			31 CAP	31 AQU	30 PIS			30 LEO

1975

JAN	FEB	MAR	APR	MAY	JUN	JUL	AUG	SEP	OCT	NOV	DEC
1 LEO	1 LIB	1 LIB	1 SAG	1 CAP	1 AQU	1 ARI	1 TAU	1 CAN	1 LEO	1 LIB	1 SCO
2 VIR	3 SCO	2 SCO	3 CAP	3 AQU	2 PIS	4 TAU	3 GEM	3 LEO	3 VIR	3 SCO	3 SAG
4 LIB	5 SAG	4 SAG	5 AQU	5 PIS	4 ARI	6 GEM	5 CAN	5 VIR	5 LIB	5 SAG	5 CAP
6 SCO	7 CAP	7 CAP	8 PIS	8 ARI	7 TAU	9 CAN	7 LEO	7 LIB	7 SCO	8 CAP	7 AQU
9 SAG	10 AQU	9 AQU	10 ARI	10 GEM	9 GEM	11 LEO	9 VIR	9 SCO	9 SAG	10 AQU	10 PIS
11 CAP	12 PIS	12 PIS	13 TAU	13 CAN	11 CAN	13 VIR	11 LIB	12 SAG	11 CAP	12 PIS	12 ARI
14 AQU	15 ARI	14 ARI	15 GEM	15 LEO	13 LEO	15 LIB	13 SCO	14 CAP	14 AQU	15 ARI	15 TAU
16 PIS	17 TAU	17 TAU	18 CAN	17 VIR	15 VIR	17 SCO	15 SAG	16 AQU	16 PIS	17 TAU	17 GEM
19 ARI	20 GEM	19 GEM	20 LEO	19 LIB	17 LIB	19 SAG	18 CAP	19 PIS	19 ARI	20 GEM	19 CAN
21 TAU	22 CAN	21 CAN	22 VIR	21 SCO	20 SCO	21 CAP	20 AQU	21 ARI	21 TAU	22 CAN	22 LEO
23 GEM	24 LEO	24 LEO	24 LIB	23 SAG	22 SAG	24 AQU	22 PIS	24 TAU	23 GEM	24 LEO	24 VIR
26 CAN	26 VIR	26 VIR	26 SCO	25 CAP	24 CAP	26 PIS	25 ARI	26 GEM	26 CAN	27 VIR	26 LIB
28 LEO	28 LIB	28 LIB	28 SAG	28 AQU	26 AQU	29 ARI	28 TAU	29 CAN	28 LEO	29 LIB	28 SCO
30 VIR		30 SCO	30 CAP	30 PIS	29 PIS	31 TAU	30 GEM	30 VIR	31 SAG
31 VIR		31 SCO		31 AQU	30 PIS		31 GEM				31 SAG

1976

JAN	FEB	MAR	APR	MAY	JUN	JUL	AUG	SEP	OCT	NOV	DEC
1 CAP	1 AQU	1 PIS	1 ARI	1 TAU	1 CAN	1 LEO	1 LIB	1 SAG	1 CAP	1 PIS	1 ARI
4 AQU	2 PIS	3 ARI	2 TAU	2 GEM	3 LEO	2 VIR	3 SCO	3 CAP	3 AQU	4 ARI	3 TAU
6 PIS	5 ARI	6 TAU	4 GEM	4 CAN	5 VIR	4 LIB	5 SAG	5 AQU	5 PIS	6 TAU	6 GEM
8 ARI	7 TAU	8 GEM	7 CAN	6 LEO	7 LIB	6 SCO	7 CAP	8 PIS	7 ARI	9 GEM	8 CAN
11 TAU	10 GEM	11 CAN	9 LEO	9 VIR	9 SCO	9 SAG	9 AQU	10 ARI	10 TAU	11 CAN	11 LEO
13 GEM	12 CAN	13 LEO	11 VIR	11 LIB	11 SAG	11 CAP	11 PIS	13 TAU	13 GEM	14 LEO	13 VIR
16 CAN	14 LEO	15 VIR	13 LIB	13 SCO	13 CAP	13 AQU	14 ARI	15 GEM	15 CAN	16 VIR	15 LIB
18 LEO	16 VIR	17 LIB	15 SCO	15 SAG	15 AQU	15 PIS	16 TAU	18 CAN	17 LEO	18 LIB	18 SCO
20 VIR	18 LIB	19 SCO	17 SAG	17 CAP	18 PIS	18 ARI	19 GEM	20 LEO	20 VIR	20 SCO	20 SAG
22 LIB	21 SCO	21 SAG	19 CAP	19 AQU	20 ARI	20 TAU	21 CAN	22 VIR	22 LIB	22 SAG	22 CAP
24 SCO	23 SAG	23 CAP	22 AQU	21 PIS	23 TAU	23 GEM	23 LEO	24 LIB	24 SCO	24 CAP	24 AQU
26 SAG	25 CAP	25 AQU	24 PIS	24 ARI	25 GEM	25 CAN	25 VIR	26 SCO	26 SAG	26 AQU	26 PIS
29 CAP	27 AQU	28 PIS	27 ARI	27 TAU	28 CAN	27 LEO	27 LIB	28 SAG	28 CAP	28 PIS	28 ARI
31 AQU	29 AQU	30 ARI	29 TAU	29 GEM	30 LEO	29 VIR	29 SCO	30 CAP	30 AQU	30 PIS	31 TAU
		31 ARI		31 CAN		31 VIR	31 SCO				

1977

JAN	FEB	MAR	APR	MAY	JUN	JUL	AUG	SEP	OCT	NOV	DEC
1 TAU	1 CAN	1 CAN	1 LEO	1 LIB	1 SCO	1 CAP	1 AQU	1 ARI	1 TAU	1 CAN	1 LEO
2 GEM	4 LEO	3 LEO	2 VIR	3 SCO	2 SAG	3 AQU	2 PIS	3 TAU	2 GEM	4 LEO	3 VIR
5 CAN	6 VIR	5 VIR	4 LIB	5 SAG	4 CAP	5 PIS	4 ARI	5 GEM	5 CAN	6 VIR	6 LIB
7 LEO	8 LIB	7 LIB	6 SCO	7 CAP	6 AQU	7 ARI	6 TAU	8 CAN	7 LEO	8 LIB	8 SCO
9 VIR	10 SCO	9 SCO	8 SAG	9 AQU	8 PIS	10 TAU	9 GEM	10 LEO	10 VIR	11 SCO	10 SAG
12 LIB	12 SAG	11 SAG	10 CAP	11 PIS	10 ARI	12 GEM	11 CAN	12 VIR	12 LIB	13 SAG	12 CAP
14 SCO	14 CAP	14 CAP	12 AQU	14 ARI	13 TAU	15 CAN	14 LEO	14 LIB	14 SCO	15 CAP	14 AQU
16 SAG	16 AQU	16 AQU	14 PIS	16 TAU	15 GEM	17 LEO	16 VIR	17 SCO	16 SAG	17 AQU	16 PIS
18 CAP	19 PIS	18 PIS	17 ARI	19 GEM	18 CAN	20 VIR	18 LIB	19 SAG	18 CAP	19 PIS	18 ARI
20 AQU	21 ARI	20 ARI	19 TAU	21 CAN	20 LEO	22 LIB	20 SCO	21 CAP	20 AQU	21 ARI	21 TAU
22 PIS	23 TAU	23 TAU	21 GEM	24 LEO	23 VIR	24 SCO	23 SAG	23 AQU	23 PIS	23 TAU	23 GEM
25 ARI	26 GEM	25 GEM	24 CAN	26 VIR	25 LIB	26 SAG	25 CAP	25 PIS	25 ARI	25 GEM	26 CAN
27 TAU	28 CAN	28 CAN	27 LEO	29 LIB	27 SCO	28 CAP	27 AQU	28 ARI	27 TAU	28 CAN	28 LEO
30 GEM		30 LEO	29 VIR	31 SCO	29 SAG	30 AQU	29 PIS	30 TAU	30 GEM	30 CAN	31 VIR
31 GEM		31 LEO			30 SAG	31 AQU	31 ARI		31 GEM		

246

Moon Ephemeris: How to Find Your Moon Sign

1978

JAN	FEB	MAR	APR	MAY	JUN	JUL	AUG	SEP	OCT	NOV	DEC
1 VIR	1 SCO	1 SCO	1 CAP	1 AQU	1 ARI	1 TAU	1 CAN	1 LEO	1 VIR	1 SCO	1 SAG
2 LIB	3 SAG	2 SAG	3 AQU	2 PIS	3 TAU	3 GEM	4 LEO	2 VIR	2 LIB	3 SAG	2 CAP
4 SCO	5 CAP	4 CAP	5 PIS	4 ARI	5 GEM	5 CAN	6 VIR	5 LIB	4 SCO	5 CAP	4 AQU
6 SAG	7 AQU	6 AQU	7 ARI	6 TAU	8 CAN	7 LEO	9 LIB	7 SCO	7 SAG	7 AQU	6 PIS
8 CAP	9 PIS	8 PIS	9 TAU	9 GEM	10 LEO	10 VIR	11 SCO	9 SAG	9 CAP	9 PIS	9 ARI
10 AQU	11 ARI	10 ARI	11 GEM	11 CAN	13 VIR	12 LIB	13 SAG	12 CAP	11 AQU	11 ARI	11 TAU
12 PIS	13 TAU	13 TAU	14 CAN	14 LEO	15 LIB	15 SCO	15 CAP	14 AQU	13 PIS	14 TAU	13 GEM
15 ARI	16 GEM	15 GEM	16 LEO	16 VIR	17 SCO	17 SAG	17 AQU	16 PIS	15 ARI	16 GEM	16 CAN
17 TAU	18 CAN	18 CAN	19 VIR	19 LIB	19 SAG	19 CAP	19 PIS	18 ARI	17 TAU	18 CAN	18 LEO
19 GEM	21 LEO	20 LEO	21 LIB	21 SCO	21 CAP	21 AQU	21 ARI	20 TAU	20 GEM	21 LEO	21 VIR
22 CAN	23 VIR	23 VIR	23 SCO	23 SAG	23 AQU	23 PIS	24 TAU	22 GEM	22 CAN	23 VIR	23 LIB
25 LEO	26 LIB	25 LIB	25 CAP	25 PIS	25 ARI	26 GEM	25 CAN	25 LEO	26 LIB	26 SCO
27 VIR	28 SCO	27 SCO	28 CAP	27 AQU	28 ARI	27 TAU	28 CAN	27 LEO	27 VIR	28 SCO	28 SAG
29 LIB		29 SAG	30 AQU	29 PIS	30 TAU	30 GEM	31 LEO	30 VIR	29 LIB	30 SAG	30 CAP
31 LIB		31 CAP				31 CAN			31 SCO		

1979

JAN	FEB	MAR	APR	MAY	JUN	JUL	AUG	SEP	OCT	NOV	DEC
1 AQU	1 ARI	1 ARI	1 GEM	1 CAN	1 LEO	1 VIR	1 SCO	1 SAG	1 AQU	1 PIS	1 TAU
3 PIS	3 TAU	4 CAN	4 LEO	2 VIR	2 LIB	3 SAG	2 CAP	2 CAP	4 PIS	2 ARI	3 GEM
5 ARI	6 GEM	5 GEM	6 LEO	6 VIR	5 LIB	5 SCO	6 CAP	4 AQU	6 ARI	4 TAU	6 CAN
7 TAU	8 CAN	7 CAN	9 VIR	9 LIB	7 SCO	7 SAG	8 AQU	6 PIS	8 TAU	6 GEM	8 LEO
9 GEM	11 LEO	10 LEO	11 LIB	11 SCO	10 SAG	9 CAP	10 PIS	8 ARI	10 GEM	8 CAN	10 VIR
12 CAN	13 VIR	13 VIR	14 SCO	13 SAG	12 CAP	11 AQU	12 ARI	10 TAU	12 CAN	11 LEO	13 LIB
14 LEO	16 LIB	15 LIB	16 SAG	15 CAP	14 AQU	13 PIS	14 TAU	12 GEM	14 LEO	13 VIR	16 SCO
17 VIR	18 SCO	17 SCO	18 CAP	18 AQU	16 PIS	15 ARI	16 GEM	15 CAN	17 VIR	16 LIB	18 SAG
19 LIB	20 SAG	20 SAG	20 AQU	20 PIS	18 ARI	17 TAU	18 CAN	17 LEO	19 LIB	18 SCO	20 CAP
22 SCO	23 CAP	22 CAP	22 PIS	22 ARI	20 TAU	20 GEM	21 LEO	20 VIR	22 SCO	20 SAG	22 AQU
24 SAG	25 AQU	24 AQU	25 ARI	24 TAU	22 GEM	22 CAN	23 VIR	22 LIB	24 SAG	23 CAP	24 PIS
26 CAP	27 PIS	26 PIS	27 TAU	26 GEM	25 CAN	25 LEO	26 LIB	25 SCO	27 CAP	25 AQU	26 ARI
28 AQU	28 PIS	28 ARI	29 GEM	28 CAN	27 LEO	27 VIR	28 SCO	27 SAG	29 AQU	27 PIS	29 TAU
30 PIS		30 TAU	30 GEM	31 LEO	30 SAG	30 LIB	31 SAG	29 CAP	31 PIS	29 ARI	31 GEM
31 PIS		31 TAU				31 LIB		30 CAP		30 ARI	

1980

JAN	FEB	MAR	APR	MAY	JUN	JUL	AUG	SEP	OCT	NOV	DEC
1 GEM	1 LEO	1 VIR	1 LIB	1 SCO	1 CAP	1 AQU	1 ARI	1 TAU	1 CAN	1 LEO	1 LIB
2 CAN	3 VIR	4 LIB	3 SCO	2 SAG	3 AQU	3 PIS	3 TAU	2 GEM	3 LEO	2 VIR	2 LIB
4 LEO	6 LIB	6 SCO	5 SAG	5 CAP	6 PIS	5 ARI	5 GEM	4 CAN	6 VIR	5 LIB	4 SCO
7 VIR	8 SCO	9 SAG	8 CAP	7 AQU	8 ARI	7 TAU	8 CAN	6 LEO	8 LIB	7 SCO	7 SAG
9 LIB	11 SAG	11 CAP	10 AQU	9 PIS	10 TAU	9 GEM	10 LEO	9 VIR	11 SCO	10 SAG	9 CAP
12 SCO	13 CAP	13 AQU	12 PIS	11 ARI	12 GEM	11 CAN	12 VIR	11 LIB	13 SAG	12 CAP	12 AQU
14 SAG	15 AQU	16 PIS	14 ARI	13 TAU	14 CAN	14 LEO	15 LIB	14 SCO	16 CAP	14 AQU	14 PIS
16 CAP	17 PIS	18 ARI	16 TAU	15 GEM	16 LEO	16 VIR	17 SCO	16 SAG	18 AQU	17 PIS	16 ARI
19 AQU	19 ARI	20 TAU	18 GEM	18 CAN	19 VIR	18 LIB	20 SAG	18 CAP	20 PIS	19 ARI	18 TAU
21 PIS	21 TAU	22 GEM	20 CAN	20 LEO	21 LIB	21 SCO	22 CAP	21 AQU	22 ARI	21 TAU	20 GEM
23 ARI	23 GEM	24 CAN	22 LEO	22 VIR	24 SCO	23 SAG	24 AQU	23 PIS	24 TAU	23 GEM	22 CAN
25 TAU	26 CAN	26 LEO	25 VIR	25 LIB	26 SAG	26 CAP	26 PIS	25 ARI	26 GEM	25 CAN	24 LEO
27 GEM	28 LEO	29 VIR	27 LIB	27 SCO	28 CAP	28 AQU	28 ARI	27 TAU	28 CAN	27 LEO	27 VIR
29 CAN	29 LEO	31 LIB	30 SCO	30 SAG	30 CAP	30 PIS	30 TAU	29 GEM	31 LEO	29 VIR	29 LIB
31 LEO				31 SAG		31 PIS	31 TAU	30 GEM		30 VIR	31 LIB

1981

JAN	FEB	MAR	APR	MAY	JUN	JUL	AUG	SEP	OCT	NOV	DEC
1 SCO	1 SAG	1 CAP	1 AQU	1 PIS	1 TAU	1 GEM	1 LEO	1 LIB	1 SCO	1 SAG	1 AQU
3 SAG	2 CAP	4 AQU	2 PIS	2 ARI	2 GEM	2 CAN	2 VIR	3 SCO	3 SAG	2 CAP	3 AQU
6 CAP	4 AQU	6 PIS	4 ARI	4 TAU	4 CAN	4 LEO	5 LIB	6 SAG	6 CAP	5 AQU	4 PIS
8 AQU	6 PIS	8 ARI	6 TAU	6 GEM	6 LEO	6 VIR	7 SCO	8 CAP	8 AQU	7 PIS	6 ARI
10 PIS	9 ARI	10 TAU	8 GEM	9 CAN	9 VIR	8 LIB	10 SAG	10 AQU	11 PIS	9 ARI	9 TAU
12 ARI	11 TAU	12 GEM	10 CAN	10 LEO	11 LIB	11 SCO	12 CAP	13 PIS	13 ARI	11 TAU	11 GEM
14 TAU	13 GEM	14 CAN	13 LEO	13 VIR	14 SCO	13 SAG	14 AQU	15 ARI	15 TAU	13 GEM	13 CAN
17 GEM	15 CAN	16 LEO	15 VIR	15 LIB	16 SAG	16 CAP	17 PIS	17 TAU	17 GEM	15 CAN	15 LEO
19 CAN	17 LEO	19 VIR	17 LIB	17 SCO	18 CAP	18 AQU	19 ARI	19 GEM	19 CAN	19 VIR	17 VIR
21 LEO	19 VIR	21 LIB	20 SCO	20 SAG	22 CAP	20 PIS	21 TAU	21 CAN	21 LEO	19 VIR	19 LIB
23 VIR	22 LIB	24 SCO	22 SAG	22 CAP	23 PIS	23 ARI	23 GEM	24 LEO	22 LIB	21 SCO
25 LIB	24 SCO	26 SAG	25 CAP	25 AQU	25 ARI	25 TAU	25 CAN	26 VIR	26 LIB	24 SCO	24 SAG
28 SCO	27 SAG	29 CAP	27 AQU	27 PIS	28 TAU	27 CAN	27 CAN	30 VIR	28 LIB	28 SCO	27 CAP
31 SAG	28 SAG	31 AQU	30 PIS	29 ARI	30 GEM	29 CAN	30 VIR	30 LIB	27 SAG	29 AQU
				31 TAU		31 LEO	31 VIR		31 SAG	30 CAP	31 PIS

1982

JAN	FEB	MAR	APR	MAY	JUN	JUL	AUG	SEP	OCT	NOV	DEC
1 PIS	1 TAU	1 TAU	1 CAN	1 LEO	1 LIB	1 SCO	1 SAG	1 AQU	1 PIS	1 TAU	1 GEM
3 ARI	3 GEM	3 GEM	3 LEO	2 VIR	3 SCO	3 SAG	2 CAP	3 PIS	3 ARI	4 GEM	3 CAN
5 TAU	5 CAN	5 CAN	5 VIR	5 LIB	6 SAG	5 CAP	4 AQU	6 ARI	5 TAU	6 CAN	5 LEO
7 GEM	7 LEO	7 LEO	8 LIB	7 SCO	8 CAP	8 AQU	7 PIS	8 TAU	7 GEM	8 LEO	7 VIR
9 CAN	10 VIR	9 VIR	10 SCO	10 SAG	11 AQU	11 PIS	9 ARI	10 GEM	9 CAN	10 VIR	9 LIB
11 LEO	12 LIB	11 LIB	12 SAG	12 CAP	13 PIS	13 ARI	12 TAU	12 CAN	11 LEO	12 LIB	12 SCO
13 VIR	14 SCO	14 SCO	15 CAP	15 AQU	16 ARI	15 TAU	14 GEM	14 LEO	14 VIR	14 SCO	14 SAG
15 LIB	17 SAG	16 SAG	17 AQU	17 PIS	18 TAU	17 GEM	16 CAN	16 VIR	16 LIB	17 SAG	16 CAP
18 SCO	19 CAP	19 CAP	20 PIS	19 ARI	20 GEM	19 CAN	18 LEO	18 LIB	18 SCO	19 CAP	19 AQU
20 SAG	22 AQU	21 AQU	22 ARI	22 TAU	22 CAN	21 LEO	20 VIR	21 SCO	20 SAG	22 AQU	22 PIS
23 CAP	24 PIS	23 PIS	24 TAU	24 GEM	24 LEO	23 VIR	23 LIB	23 SAG	23 CAP	24 PIS	24 ARI
25 AQU	26 ARI	26 ARI	26 GEM	26 CAN	26 VIR	25 LIB	25 SCO	28 AQU	25 AQU	27 ARI	26 TAU
28 PIS	28 TAU	28 TAU	28 CAN	28 LEO	28 LIB	28 SCO	28 SAG	30 AQU	30 ARI	29 TAU	28 GEM
30 ARI		30 GEM	30 LEO	30 VIR	30 SCO	30 SAG	29 CAP		30 ARI	30 TAU	30 CAN
31 ARI		31 GEM		31 VIR		31 SAG	31 CAP				31 CAN

247

Healing Mind, Body, Spirit

1983

JAN	FEB	MAR	APR	MAY	JUN	JUL	AUG	SEP	OCT	NOV	DEC
2 VIR	1 LIB	2 SCO	1 SAG	1 CAP	2 PIS	2 ARI	1 TAU	1 CAN	1 LEO	1 LIB	1 SCO
4 LIB	3 SCO	5 SAG	3 CAP	3 AQU	5 ARI	4 TAU	3 GEM	3 LEO	3 VIR	3 SCO	3 SAG
7 SCO	5 SAG	7 CAP	6 AQU	6 PIS	7 TAU	7 GEM	5 CAN	5 VIR	5 LIB	6 SAG	5 CAP
9 SAG	8 CAP	10 AQU	8 PIS	8 ARI	9 GEM	9 CAN	7 LEO	7 LIB	7 SCO	8 CAP	8 AQU
12 CAP	10 AQU	12 PIS	11 ARI	11 TAU	11 CAN	11 LEO	9 VIR	10 SCO	9 SAG	10 AQU	10 PIS
14 AQU	13 PIS	15 ARI	13 TAU	13 GEM	13 LEO	13 VIR	11 LIB	12 SAG	11 CAP	13 PIS	13 ARI
17 PIS	15 ARI	17 TAU	15 GEM	15 CAN	15 VIR	15 LIB	13 SCO	14 CAP	14 AQU	15 ARI	15 TAU
19 ARI	18 TAU	19 GEM	18 CAN	17 LEO	17 LIB	17 SCO	15 SAG	17 AQU	16 PIS	18 TAU	17 GEM
21 TAU	20 GEM	21 CAN	20 LEO	19 VIR	20 SCO	19 SAG	18 CAP	19 PIS	19 ARI	20 GEM	20 CAN
24 GEM	22 CAN	23 LEO	22 VIR	21 LIB	22 SAG	22 CAP	20 AQU	22 ARI	21 TAU	22 CAN	22 LEO
26 CAN	24 LEO	26 VIR	24 LIB	23 SCO	24 CAP	24 AQU	23 PIS	24 TAU	24 GEM	24 LEO	24 VIR
28 LEO	26 VIR	28 LIB	26 SCO	26 SAG	27 AQU	27 PIS	25 ARI	26 GEM	26 CAN	26 VIR	28 LIB
30 VIR	28 LIB	30 SCO	28 SAG	28 CAP	29 PIS	29 ARI	28 TAU	29 CAN	28 LEO	29 LIB	28 SCO
				31 AQU			30 GEM		30 VIR		30 SAG

1984

JAN	FEB	MAR	APR	MAY	JUN	JUL	AUG	SEP	OCT	NOV	DEC
2 CAP	3 PIS	1 PIS	2 SAU	2 GEM	1 CAN	2 VIR	3 SCO	1 SAG	1 CAP	2 PIS	1 ARI
4 AQU	5 ARI	4 ARI	5 GEM	4 CAN	3 LEO	4 LIB	5 SAG	3 CAP	3 AQU	4 ARI	4 TAU
6 PIS	8 TAU	6 TAU	7 CAN	6 LEO	5 VIR	6 SCO	7 CAP	6 AQU	5 PIS	7 TAU	6 GEM
9 ARI	10 GEM	8 GEM	9 LEO	9 VIR	7 LIB	9 SAG	9 AQU	8 PIS	8 ARI	9 GEM	9 CAN
11 TAU	12 CAN	11 CAN	11 VIR	11 LIB	9 SCO	11 CAP	12 PIS	11 ARI	10 TAU	12 CAN	11 LEO
14 GEM	15 LEO	13 LEO	13 LIB	13 SCO	11 SAG	13 AQU	14 ARI	13 TAU	13 GEM	14 LEO	13 VIR
16 CAN	17 VIR	15 VIR	15 SCO	15 SAG	13 CAP	16 PIS	17 TAU	16 GEM	15 CAN	16 VIR	15 LIB
18 LEO	19 LIB	17 LIB	17 SAG	17 CAP	16 AQU	18 ARI	19 GEM	18 CAN	18 LEO	18 LIB	17 SCO
20 VIR	21 SCO	19 SCO	20 CAP	19 AQU	18 PIS	21 TAU	22 CAN	20 LEO	20 VIR	20 SCO	20 SAG
22 LIB	23 SAG	21 SAG	22 AQU	22 PIS	21 ARI	23 GEM	24 LEO	22 VIR	22 LIB	22 SAG	22 CAP
24 SCO	25 CAP	23 CAP	25 PIS	24 ARI	23 TAU	25 CAN	26 VIR	24 LIB	24 SCO	24 CAP	24 AQU
26 SAG	28 AQU	26 AQU	27 ARI	27 TAU	26 GEM	27 LEO	28 LIB	26 SCO	26 SAG	27 AQU	26 PIS
29 CAP		28 PIS	30 TAU	29 GEM	28 CAN	29 VIR	30 SCO	28 SAG	28 CAP	29 PIS	29 ARI
31 AQU		31 ARI			30 LEO	31 LIB			30 AQU		31 TAU

1985

JAN	FEB	MAR	APR	MAY	JUN	JUL	AUG	SEP	OCT	NOV	DEC
3 GEM	2 CAN	1 CAN	2 VIR	1 LIB	2 SAG	1 CAP	2 PIS	1 ARI	3 GEM	2 CAN	1 LEO
5 CAN	4 LEO	3 LEO	4 LIB	3 SCO	4 CAP	3 AQU	4 ARI	3 TAU	5 CAN	4 LEO	4 VIR
7 LEO	6 VIR	5 VIR	6 SCO	5 SAG	6 AQU	5 PIS	7 TAU	6 GEM	8 LEO	6 VIR	6 LIB
9 VIR	8 LIB	7 LIB	8 SAG	7 CAP	8 PIS	8 ARI	9 GEM	8 CAN	10 VIR	9 LIB	8 SCO
12 LIB	10 SCO	9 SCO	10 CAP	9 AQU	11 ARI	10 TAU	12 CAN	10 LEO	12 LIB	11 SCO	10 SAG
14 SCO	12 SAG	11 SAG	12 AQU	12 PIS	13 TAU	13 GEM	14 LEO	12 VIR	14 SCO	13 SAG	12 CAP
16 SAG	14 CAP	14 CAP	14 PIS	14 ARI	16 GEM	15 CAN	16 VIR	15 LIB	16 SAG	15 CAP	14 AQU
18 CAP	17 AQU	16 AQU	17 ARI	17 TAU	18 CAN	18 LEO	18 LIB	17 SCO	18 CAP	17 AQU	16 PIS
20 AQU	19 PIS	18 PIS	20 TAU	19 GEM	20 LEO	20 VIR	20 SCO	20 AQU	19 PIS	19 ARI
23 PIS	21 ARI	21 ARI	22 GEM	22 CAN	23 VIR	22 LIB	22 SAG	21 CAP	23 PIS	21 ARI	21 TAU
25 ARI	24 TAU	23 TAU	25 CAN	24 LEO	25 LIB	25 SCO	25 CAP	23 AQU	25 ARI	24 TAU	24 GEM
28 TAU	27 GEM	26 GEM	27 LEO	26 VIR	27 SCO	26 SAG	27 AQU	25 PIS	28 TAU	26 GEM	26 CAN
30 GEM		28 CAN	29 VIR	29 LIB	29 SAG	28 CAP	29 PIS	28 ARI	30 GEM	29 CAN	29 LEO
		31 LEO		31 SCO		31 AQU		30 TAU			31 VIR

1986

JAN	FEB	MAR	APR	MAY	JUN	JUL	AUG	SEP	OCT	NOV	DEC
2 LIB	1 SCO	2 SAG	2 AQU	2 PIS	3 TAU	3 GEM	2 CAN	3 VIR	2 LIB	1 SCO	2 CAP
4 SCO	3 SAG	4 CAP	5 PIS	4 ARI	5 GEM	5 CAN	4 LEO	5 LIB	4 SCO	3 SAG	4 AQU
6 SAG	5 CAP	6 AQU	7 ARI	7 TAU	8 CAN	8 LEO	6 VIR	7 SCO	7 SAG	5 CAP	6 PIS
8 CAP	7 AQU	8 PIS	9 TAU	9 GEM	11 LEO	10 VIR	9 LIB	9 SAG	9 CAP	7 AQU	9 ARI
11 AQU	9 PIS	11 ARI	12 GEM	12 CAN	13 VIR	12 LIB	11 SCO	11 CAP	11 AQU	9 PIS	11 TAU
13 PIS	11 ARI	13 TAU	14 CAN	14 LEO	15 LIB	15 SCO	13 SAG	14 AQU	13 PIS	11 ARI	14 GEM
15 ARI	14 TAU	16 GEM	17 LEO	17 VIR	17 SCO	17 SAG	15 CAP	15 PIS	15 ARI	14 TAU	16 CAN
17 TAU	16 GEM	18 CAN	19 VIR	19 LIB	19 SAG	19 CAP	17 AQU	18 ARI	18 TAU	16 GEM	19 LEO
20 GEM	19 CAN	21 LEO	21 LIB	21 SCO	21 CAP	21 AQU	19 PIS	20 TAU	20 GEM	19 CAN	21 VIR
22 CAN	21 LEO	23 VIR	24 SCO	23 SAG	23 AQU	23 PIS	22 ARI	23 GEM	23 CAN	21 LEO	24 LIB
25 LEO	24 VIR	25 LIB	26 SAG	25 CAP	26 PIS	25 ARI	24 TAU	25 CAN	25 LEO	24 VIR	26 SCO
27 VIR	26 LIB	27 SCO	28 CAP	27 AQU	28 ARI	28 TAU	26 GEM	28 LEO	27 VIR	26 LIB	28 SAG
29 LIB	28 SCO	29 SAG	30 AQU	29 PIS	30 TAU	30 GEM	29 CAN	30 VIR	30 LIB	28 SCO	30 CAP
		31 CAP		31 ARI			31 LEO			30 SAG	

1987

JAN	FEB	MAR	APR	MAY	JUN	JUL	AUG	SEP	OCT	NOV	DEC
1 AQU	1 ARI	1 ARI	2 GEM	2 CAN	3 VIR	3 LIB	1 SCO	2 CAP	1 AQU	2 ARI	1 TAU
3 PIS	4 TAU	3 TAU	4 CAN	4 LEO	5 LIB	5 SCO	4 SAG	4 AQU	3 PIS	4 TAU	4 GEM
5 ARI	6 GEM	5 GEM	7 LEO	7 VIR	8 SCO	7 SAG	6 CAP	6 PIS	6 ARI	6 GEM	6 CAN
7 TAU	9 CAN	8 CAN	9 VIR	9 LIB	10 SAG	9 CAP	8 AQU	8 ARI	8 TAU	9 CAN	8 LEO
10 GEM	11 LEO	10 LEO	12 LIB	11 SCO	12 CAP	11 AQU	10 PIS	10 TAU	10 GEM	11 LEO	11 VIR
12 CAN	14 VIR	13 VIR	14 SCO	13 SAG	14 AQU	13 PIS	12 ARI	14 TAU	13 CAN	14 VIR	14 LIB
15 LEO	16 LIB	15 LIB	16 SAG	15 CAP	16 PIS	15 ARI	14 TAU	15 CAN	15 LEO	16 LIB	16 SCO
17 VIR	18 SCO	18 SCO	18 CAP	17 AQU	18 ARI	18 TAU	16 GEM	17 VIR	17 VIR	18 SCO	18 SAG
20 LIB	21 SAG	20 SAG	20 AQU	20 PIS	20 TAU	20 GEM	19 CAN	20 VIR	20 LIB	21 SAG	20 CAP
22 SCO	23 CAP	22 CAP	22 PIS	22 ARI	23 GEM	22 CAN	21 LEO	22 LIB	22 SCO	23 CAP	22 AQU
24 SAG	25 AQU	24 AQU	25 ARI	24 TAU	25 CAN	25 LEO	24 VIR	25 SCO	24 SAG	25 AQU	24 PIS
26 CAP	27 PIS	26 PIS	27 TAU	26 GEM	28 LEO	27 VIR	26 LIB	27 SAG	26 CAP	27 PIS	26 ARI
28 AQU		28 ARI	29 GEM	29 CAN	30 VIR	30 LIB	29 SCO	29 CAP	29 AQU	29 ARI	29 TAU
30 PIS		30 TAU		31 LEO			31 SAG		31 PIS		31 GEM

248

Moon Ephemeris: How to Find Your Moon Sign

1988

JAN	FEB	MAR	APR	MAY	JUN	JUL	AUG	SEP	OCT	NOV	DEC
2 CAN	1 LEO	2 VIR	1 LIB	3 SAG	1 CAP	1 AQU	1 ARI	2 GEM	1 CAN	2 VIR	2 LIB
5 LEO	4 VIR	4 LIB	3 SCO	5 CAP	3 AQU	3 PIS	3 TAU	4 CAN	4 LEO	5 LIB	5 SCO
7 VIR	6 LIB	7 SCO	5 SAG	7 AQU	5 PIS	5 ARI	5 GEM	6 LEO	6 VIR	7 SCO	7 SAG
10 LIB	9 SCO	9 SAG	8 CAP	9 PIS	8 ARI	7 TAU	8 CAN	9 VIR	9 LIB	10 SAG	9 CAP
12 SCO	11 SAG	11 CAP	10 AQU	11 ARI	10 TAU	9 GEM	10 LEO	11 LIB	11 SCO	12 CAP	12 AQU
15 SAG	13 CAP	14 AQU	12 PIS	13 TAU	12 GEM	11 CAN	13 VIR	14 SCO	14 SAG	14 AQU	14 PIS
17 CAP	15 AQU	16 PIS	14 ARI	16 GEM	14 CAN	14 LEO	15 LIB	16 SAG	16 CAP	17 PIS	16 ARI
19 AQU	17 PIS	18 ARI	16 TAU	18 CAN	17 LEO	16 VIR	18 SCO	19 CAP	18 AQU	19 ARI	18 TAU
21 PIS	19 ARI	20 TAU	18 GEM	20 LEO	19 VIR	19 LIB	20 SAG	21 AQU	20 PIS	21 TAU	20 GEM
23 ARI	21 TAU	22 GEM	20 CAN	23 VIR	21 LIB	21 SCO	22 CAP	23 PIS	22 ARI	23 GEM	22 CAN
25 TAU	23 GEM	24 CAN	23 LEO	25 LIB	24 SCO	24 SAG	24 AQU	25 ARI	24 TAU	25 CAN	25 LEO
27 GEM	26 CAN	27 LEO	25 VIR	28 SCO	26 SAG	26 CAP	26 PIS	27 TAU	26 GEM	27 LEO	27 VIR
30 CAN	28 LEO	29 VIR	28 LIB	30 SAG	29 CAP	28 AQU	28 ARI	29 GEM	29 CAN	30 VIR	30 LIB
			30 SCO			30 PIS	30 TAU		31 LEO		

1989

JAN	FEB	MAR	APR	MAY	JUN	JUL	AUG	SEP	OCT	NOV	DEC
1 SCO	2 CAP	2 CAP	2 PIS	2 ARI	2 GEM	2 CAN	3 VIR	1 LIB	1 SCO	2 CAP	2 AQU
4 SAG	4 AQU	4 AQU	4 ARI	4 TAU	4 CAN	4 LEO	5 LIB	4 SCO	4 SAG	5 AQU	4 PIS
6 CAP	6 PIS	6 PIS	6 TAU	6 GEM	7 LEO	6 VIR	8 SCO	6 SAG	6 CAP	7 PIS	7 ARI
8 AQU	8 ARI	8 ARI	8 GEM	8 CAN	9 VIR	9 LIB	10 SAG	9 CAP	9 AQU	9 ARI	9 TAU
10 PIS	11 TAU	10 TAU	11 CAN	10 LEO	11 LIB	11 SCO	12 CAP	11 AQU	11 PIS	11 TAU	11 GEM
12 ARI	13 GEM	12 GEM	13 LEO	13 VIR	14 SCO	14 SAG	15 AQU	13 PIS	13 ARI	13 GEM	13 CAN
14 TAU	15 CAN	14 CAN	15 VIR	15 LIB	16 SAG	16 CAP	17 PIS	15 ARI	15 TAU	15 CAN	15 LEO
16 GEM	17 LEO	17 LEO	18 LIB	18 SCO	19 CAP	19 AQU	19 ARI	17 TAU	17 GEM	17 LEO	17 VIR
19 CAN	20 VIR	19 VIR	20 SCO	20 SAG	21 AQU	21 PIS	21 TAU	19 GEM	19 CAN	20 VIR	19 LIB
21 LEO	22 LIB	22 LIB	23 SAG	22 CAP	23 PIS	23 ARI	23 GEM	21 CAN	21 LEO	22 LIB	22 SCO
23 VIR	25 SCO	24 SCO	25 CAP	25 AQU	25 ARI	25 TAU	25 CAN	24 LEO	23 VIR	25 SCO	24 SAG
26 LIB	27 SAG	27 SAG	28 AQU	27 PIS	27 TAU	27 GEM	28 LEO	26 VIR	26 LIB	27 SAG	27 CAP
29 SCO		29 CAP	30 PIS	29 ARI	29 GEM	29 CAN	30 VIR	29 LIB	28 SCO	30 CAP	29 AQU
31 SAG		31 AQU		31 TAU		31 LEO			31 SAG		

1990

JAN	FEB	MAR	APR	MAY	JUN	JUL	AUG	SEP	OCT	NOV	DEC
1 PIS	1 TAU	2 GEM	1 CAN	3 VIR	1 LIB	1 SCO	2 CAP	1 AQU	1 PIS	2 TAU	1 GEM
3 ARI	3 GEM	5 CAN	3 LEO	5 LIB	4 SCO	4 SAG	5 AQU	3 PIS	3 ARI	4 GEM	3 CAN
5 TAU	5 CAN	7 LEO	5 VIR	8 SCO	6 SAG	6 CAP	7 PIS	6 ARI	5 TAU	6 CAN	5 LEO
7 GEM	8 LEO	9 VIR	8 LIB	10 SAG	9 CAP	9 AQU	9 ARI	8 TAU	7 GEM	8 LEO	7 VIR
9 CAN	10 VIR	12 LIB	10 SCO	13 CAP	11 AQU	11 PIS	11 TAU	10 GEM	9 CAN	10 VIR	10 LIB
11 LEO	12 LIB	14 SCO	13 SAG	15 AQU	14 PIS	13 ARI	14 GEM	12 CAN	11 LEO	12 LIB	12 SCO
13 VIR	15 SCO	16 SAG	15 CAP	17 PIS	16 ARI	15 TAU	16 CAN	14 LEO	14 VIR	15 SCO	15 SAG
16 LIB	17 SAG	19 CAP	18 AQU	19 ARI	18 TAU	17 GEM	18 LEO	16 VIR	16 LIB	18 SCO	17 CAP
18 SCO	20 CAP	21 AQU	20 PIS	21 TAU	20 GEM	20 CAN	20 VIR	19 LIB	18 SCO	20 CAP	19 AQU
21 SAG	22 AQU	24 PIS	22 ARI	24 GEM	22 CAN	22 LEO	22 LIB	21 SCO	21 SAG	22 AQU	22 PIS
23 CAP	24 PIS	26 ARI	24 TAU	26 CAN	24 LEO	24 VIR	25 SCO	24 SAG	23 CAP	25 PIS	24 ARI
26 AQU	26 ARI	28 TAU	26 GEM	28 LEO	26 VIR	26 LIB	27 SAG	26 CAP	26 AQU	27 ARI	26 TAU
28 PIS	28 TAU	30 GEM	28 CAN	30 VIR	29 LIB	28 SCO	30 CAP	29 AQU	28 PIS	29 TAU	28 GEM
30 ARI			30 LEO			31 SAG			30 ARI		30 CAN

1991

JAN	FEB	MAR	APR	MAY	JUN	JUL	AUG	SEP	OCT	NOV	DEC
1 LEO	2 LIB	2 LIB	3 SAG	2 CAP	1 AQU	1 PIS	2 TAU	3 CAN	2 LEO	2 LIB	2 SCO
4 VIR	4 SCO	4 SCO	5 CAP	5 AQU	4 PIS	3 ARI	4 GEM	5 LEO	4 VIR	5 SCO	4 SAG
6 LIB	7 SAG	6 SAG	8 AQU	7 PIS	6 ARI	6 TAU	6 CAN	7 VIR	6 LIB	7 SAG	7 CAP
8 SCO	9 CAP	9 CAP	10 PIS	10 ARI	8 TAU	8 GEM	8 LEO	9 LIB	8 SCO	10 CAP	9 AQU
11 SAG	12 AQU	11 AQU	12 ARI	12 TAU	10 GEM	10 CAN	10 VIR	11 SCO	11 SAG	12 AQU	12 PIS
13 CAP	14 PIS	14 PIS	15 TAU	14 GEM	12 CAN	12 LEO	12 LIB	13 SAG	13 CAP	15 PIS	14 ARI
16 AQU	17 ARI	16 ARI	17 GEM	16 CAN	14 LEO	14 VIR	15 SCO	16 CAP	16 AQU	17 ARI	17 TAU
18 PIS	19 TAU	18 TAU	19 CAN	18 LEO	16 VIR	16 LIB	17 SAG	18 AQU	18 PIS	19 TAU	19 GEM
20 ARI	21 GEM	20 GEM	21 LEO	20 VIR	19 LIB	18 SCO	20 CAP	21 PIS	21 ARI	21 GEM	21 CAN
23 TAU	23 CAN	22 CAN	23 VIR	22 LIB	21 SCO	21 SAG	23 AQU	23 ARI	23 TAU	23 CAN	23 LEO
25 GEM	25 LEO	25 LEO	25 LIB	25 SCO	23 SAG	23 CAP	25 PIS	25 TAU	25 GEM	25 LEO	25 VIR
27 CAN	27 VIR	27 VIR	28 SCO	27 SAG	26 CAP	26 AQU	28 ARI	28 GEM	27 CAN	28 VIR	27 LIB
29 LEO		29 LIB	30 SAG	30 CAP	29 AQU	28 PIS	30 TAU	29 CAN	29 LEO	30 LIB	29 SCO
31 VIR		31 SCO				31 ARI	31 GEM		31 VIR		

1992

JAN	FEB	MAR	APR	MAY	JUN	JUL	AUG	SEP	OCT	NOV	DEC
1 SAG	2 AQU	3 PIS	1 ARI	1 TAU	2 CAN	1 LEO	2 LIB	2 SAG	2 CAP	1 AQU	1 PIS
3 CAP	4 PIS	5 ARI	4 TAU	3 GEM	4 LEO	3 VIR	4 SCO	5 CAP	5 AQU	3 PIS	3 ARI
6 AQU	7 ARI	8 TAU	6 GEM	5 CAN	6 VIR	5 LIB	6 SAG	7 AQU	7 PIS	6 ARI	6 TAU
8 PIS	9 TAU	10 GEM	8 CAN	8 LEO	8 LIB	7 SCO	8 CAP	10 PIS	10 ARI	8 TAU	8 GEM
11 ARI	12 GEM	12 CAN	10 LEO	10 VIR	10 SCO	10 SAG	11 AQU	12 ARI	12 TAU	11 GEM	10 CAN
13 TAU	14 CAN	14 LEO	12 VIR	12 LIB	13 SAG	12 CAP	13 PIS	15 TAU	14 GEM	13 CAN	12 LEO
15 GEM	16 LEO	16 VIR	15 LIB	14 SCO	15 CAP	15 AQU	16 ARI	17 GEM	17 CAN	15 LEO	14 VIR
17 CAN	18 VIR	18 LIB	17 SCO	17 SAG	17 AQU	17 PIS	18 TAU	19 CAN	19 LEO	17 VIR	16 LIB
19 LEO	20 LIB	20 SCO	19 SAG	19 CAP	20 PIS	20 ARI	21 GEM	21 LEO	21 VIR	19 LIB	19 SCO
21 VIR	22 SCO	23 SAG	21 CAP	21 AQU	22 ARI	22 TAU	23 CAN	23 VIR	23 LIB	21 SCO	21 SAG
23 LIB	24 SAG	25 CAP	24 AQU	24 PIS	25 TAU	24 GEM	25 LEO	25 LIB	25 SCO	23 SAG	23 CAP
25 SCO	27 CAP	27 AQU	26 PIS	26 ARI	27 GEM	27 CAN	27 VIR	28 SCO	27 SAG	26 CAP	26 AQU
28 SAG	29 AQU	30 PIS	29 ARI	28 TAU	29 CAN	29 LEO	29 LIB	30 SAG	29 CAP	28 AQU	28 PIS
30 CAP				31 GEM		31 VIR	31 SCO				31 ARI

249

~ *Healing Mind, Body, Spirit*

1993

JAN	FEB	MAR	APR	MAY	JUN	JUL	AUG	SEP	OCT	NOV	DEC
2 TAU	1 GEM	2 CAN	1 LEO	2 LIB	1 SCO	2 CAP	1 AQU	2 ARI	2 TAU	1 GEM	3 LEO
4 GEM	3 CAN	5 LEO	3 VIR	4 SCO	3 SAG	5 AQU	3 PIS	5 TAU	4 GEM	3 CAN	5 VIR
7 CAN	5 LEO	7 VIR	5 LIB	6 SAG	5 CAP	7 PIS	6 ARI	7 GEM	7 CAN	5 LEO	7 LIB
9 LEO	7 VIR	9 LIB	7 SCO	9 CAP	7 AQU	10 ARI	8 TAU	10 CAN	9 LEO	8 VIR	9 SCO
11 VIR	9 LIB	11 SCO	9 SAG	11 AQU	10 PIS	12 TAU	11 GEM	12 LEO	11 VIR	10 LIB	11 SAG
13 LIB	11 SCO	13 SAG	11 CAP	13 PIS	12 ARI	15 GEM	14 CAN	14 VIR	13 LIB	12 SCO	13 CAP
15 SCO	13 SAG	15 CAP	14 AQU	16 ARI	15 TAU	17 CAN	15 LEO	16 LIB	15 SCO	15 SAG	15 AQU
17 SAG	16 CAP	17 AQU	16 PIS	18 TAU	17 GEM	19 LEO	17 VIR	18 SCO	17 SAG	17 CAP	18 PIS
19 CAP	18 AQU	20 PIS	19 ARI	21 GEM	19 CAN	21 VIR	19 LIB	21 SCO	19 CAP	20 PIS	20 ARI
22 AQU	21 PIS	22 ARI	21 TAU	23 CAN	22 LEO	23 LIB	21 SCO	22 CAP	22 AQU	20 PIS	23 TAU
24 PIS	23 ARI	25 TAU	24 GEM	26 LEO	24 VIR	25 SCO	24 SAG	24 AQU	24 PIS	23 ARI	25 GEM
27 ARI	26 TAU	27 GEM	26 CAN	28 VIR	26 LIB	27 SAG	26 CAP	27 PIS	27 ARI	26 TAU	28 CAN
29 TAU	28 GEM	30 CAN	28 LEO	30 LIB	28 SCO	30 CAP	28 AQU	29 ARI	29 TAU	28 GEM	30 LEO
			30 VIR		30 SAG	31 PIS				30 CAN	

1994

JAN	FEB	MAR	APR	MAY	JUN	JUL	AUG	SEP	OCT	NOV	DEC
1 VIR	2 SCO	1 SCO	1 CAP	1 AQU	2 ARI	2 TAU	1 GEM	2 LEO	2 VIR	2 SCO	2 SAG
3 LIB	4 SAG	3 SAG	4 AQU	3 PIS	5 TAU	4 GEM	3 CAN	4 VIR	4 LIB	4 SAG	4 CAP
5 SCO	6 CAP	5 CAP	6 PIS	6 ARI	7 GEM	7 CAN	5 LEO	6 LIB	6 SCO	6 CAP	6 AQU
8 SAG	8 AQU	7 AQU	9 ARI	8 TAU	10 CAN	9 LEO	8 VIR	8 SCO	8 SAG	8 AQU	8 PIS
10 CAP	11 PIS	10 PIS	11 TAU	11 GEM	12 LEO	12 VIR	10 LIB	10 SAG	10 CAP	11 PIS	10 ARI
12 AQU	13 ARI	12 ARI	14 GEM	13 CAN	14 VIR	14 LIB	12 SCO	13 CAP	12 AQU	13 ARI	13 TAU
14 PIS	16 TAU	15 TAU	16 CAN	16 LEO	16 LIB	16 SCO	14 SAG	15 AQU	14 PIS	15 TAU	15 GEM
17 ARI	18 GEM	17 GEM	18 LEO	18 VIR	19 SCO	18 SAG	16 CAP	17 PIS	17 ARI	18 GEM	18 CAN
19 TAU	20 CAN	20 CAN	21 VIR	20 LIB	21 SAG	20 CAP	18 AQU	19 ARI	19 TAU	20 CAN	20 LEO
22 GEM	23 LEO	22 LEO	23 LIB	22 SCO	23 CAP	22 AQU	21 PIS	22 TAU	22 GEM	23 LEO	23 VIR
24 CAN	25 VIR	24 VIR	25 SCO	24 SAG	25 AQU	24 PIS	23 ARI	24 GEM	24 CAN	25 VIR	25 LIB
26 LEO	27 LIB	26 LIB	27 SAG	26 CAP	27 PIS	27 ARI	26 TAU	27 CAN	27 LEO	28 LIB	27 SCO
28 VIR		28 SCO	29 CAP	28 AQU	29 ARI	29 TAU	28 GEM	29 LEO	29 VIR	30 SCO	29 SAG
31 LIB		30 SAG		31 PIS			31 CAN		31 LIB		31 CAP

1995

JAN	FEB	MAR	APR	MAY	JUN	JUL	AUG	SEP	OCT	NOV	DEC
2 AQU	1 PIS	2 ARI	1 TAU	1 GEM	2 LEO	2 VIR	3 SCO	1 SAG	3 CAP	1 PIS	3 TAU
4 PIS	3 ARI	5 TAU	3 GEM	3 CAN	5 VIR	4 LIB	5 SAG	3 CAP	5 PIS	3 ARI	5 GEM
7 ARI	5 TAU	7 GEM	6 CAN	6 LEO	7 LIB	6 SCO	7 CAP	5 AQU	7 ARI	5 TAU	8 CAN
9 TAU	8 GEM	10 CAN	8 LEO	8 VIR	9 SCO	8 SAG	9 AQU	7 PIS	9 TAU	8 GEM	10 LEO
12 GEM	10 CAN	12 LEO	11 VIR	10 LIB	11 SAG	10 CAP	11 PIS	9 ARI	12 GEM	10 CAN	13 VIR
14 CAN	13 LEO	14 VIR	13 LIB	13 SCO	13 CAP	12 AQU	13 ARI	12 TAU	14 CAN	13 LEO	15 LIB
16 LEO	15 VIR	17 LIB	15 SCO	15 SAG	15 AQU	14 PIS	15 TAU	14 GEM	17 LEO	15 VIR	17 SCO
19 VIR	17 LIB	19 SCO	17 SAG	17 CAP	17 PIS	17 ARI	18 GEM	17 CAN	19 VIR	18 LIB	19 SAG
21 LIB	19 SCO	21 SAG	19 CAP	19 AQU	19 ARI	19 TAU	20 CAN	19 LEO	21 LIB	20 SCO	21 CAP
23 SCO	22 SAG	23 CAP	21 AQU	21 PIS	22 TAU	22 GEM	23 LEO	22 VIR	23 SCO	22 SAG	23 AQU
25 SAG	24 CAP	25 AQU	24 PIS	23 ARI	24 GEM	24 CAN	25 VIR	24 LIB	26 SAG	24 CAP	25 PIS
27 CAP	26 AQU	27 PIS	26 ARI	26 TAU	27 CAN	27 LEO	28 LIB	26 SCO	28 CAP	26 AQU	28 ARI
30 AQU	28 PIS	30 ARI	28 TAU	28 GEM	29 LEO	29 VIR	30 SCO	28 SAG	30 AQU	28 PIS	30 TAU
				31 CAN		31 LIB		30 CAP		30 ARI	

1996

JAN	FEB	MAR	APR	MAY	JUN	JUL	AUG	SEP	OCT	NOV	DEC
1 GEM	3 LEO	1 LEO	2 LIB	2 SCO	2 CAP	2 AQU	2 ARI	1 TAU	3 CAN	2 LEO	2 VIR
4 CAN	5 VIR	3 VIR	4 SCO	4 SAG	4 AQU	4 PIS	4 TAU	3 GEM	5 LEO	4 VIR	4 LIB
6 LEO	8 LIB	6 LIB	6 SAG	6 CAP	6 PIS	6 ARI	7 GEM	6 CAN	8 VIR	7 LIB	6 SCO
9 VIR	10 SCO	8 SCO	9 CAP	9 AQU	9 ARI	8 TAU	9 CAN	8 LEO	10 LIB	9 SCO	8 SAG
11 LIB	12 SAG	10 SAG	11 AQU	10 PIS	11 TAU	11 GEM	11 LEO	11 VIR	13 SCO	11 SAG	11 CAP
14 SCO	14 CAP	13 CAP	13 PIS	12 ARI	14 GEM	13 CAN	14 VIR	13 LIB	15 SAG	13 CAP	13 AQU
16 SAG	16 AQU	15 AQU	15 ARI	15 TAU	16 CAN	16 LEO	17 LIB	15 SCO	17 CAP	16 AQU	15 PIS
18 CAP	18 PIS	17 PIS	17 TAU	17 GEM	19 LEO	19 VIR	19 SCO	17 SAG	19 AQU	18 PIS	17 ARI
20 AQU	20 ARI	19 ARI	20 GEM	19 CAN	21 VIR	21 LIB	21 SAG	20 CAP	21 PIS	20 ARI	19 TAU
22 PIS	23 TAU	21 TAU	22 CAN	22 LEO	24 LIB	23 SCO	24 CAP	21 AQU	23 ARI	22 TAU	22 GEM
24 ARI	25 GEM	23 GEM	25 LEO	25 VIR	26 SCO	25 SAG	26 AQU	24 PIS	26 TAU	24 GEM	24 CAN
26 TAU	27 CAN	26 CAN	27 VIR	27 LIB	28 SAG	27 CAP	28 PIS	26 ARI	28 GEM	27 CAN	26 LEO
29 GEM		28 LEO	30 LIB	29 SCO	30 CAP	30 AQU	30 ARI	28 TAU	30 CAN	29 LEO	29 VIR
31 CAN		31 VIR		31 SAG				30 GEM			31 LIB

1997

JAN	FEB	MAR	APR	MAY	JUN	JUL	AUG	SEP	OCT	NOV	DEC
3 SCO	1 SAG	1 SAG	1 AQU	1 PIS	1 TAU	1 GEM	2 LEO	3 LIB	3 SCO	1 SAG	1 CAP
5 SAG	4 CAP	3 CAP	4 PIS	3 ARI	4 GEM	3 CAN	4 VIR	6 SCO	5 SAG	4 CAP	3 AQU
7 CAP	6 AQU	5 AQU	6 ARI	5 TAU	6 CAN	6 LEO	7 LIB	8 SAG	8 CAP	6 AQU	5 PIS
9 AQU	8 PIS	7 PIS	8 TAU	7 GEM	8 LEO	8 VIR	9 SCO	10 CAP	10 AQU	8 PIS	8 ARI
11 PIS	10 ARI	9 ARI	10 GEM	9 CAN	11 VIR	10 LIB	12 SAG	12 AQU	12 PIS	10 ARI	10 TAU
13 ARI	12 TAU	11 TAU	12 CAN	12 LEO	13 LIB	13 SCO	14 CAP	15 PIS	14 ARI	12 TAU	12 GEM
15 TAU	14 GEM	13 GEM	14 LEO	14 VIR	16 SCO	15 SAG	16 AQU	17 ARI	16 TAU	14 GEM	14 CAN
18 GEM	16 CAN	16 CAN	17 VIR	17 LIB	18 SAG	18 CAP	18 PIS	19 TAU	18 GEM	17 CAN	16 LEO
20 CAN	19 LEO	18 LEO	19 LIB	19 SCO	20 CAP	20 AQU	20 ARI	21 GEM	20 CAN	19 LEO	19 VIR
23 LEO	21 VIR	21 VIR	22 SCO	22 SAG	22 AQU	22 PIS	22 TAU	23 CAN	23 LEO	21 VIR	21 LIB
25 VIR	24 LIB	23 LIB	24 SAG	24 CAP	24 PIS	24 ARI	24 GEM	25 LEO	25 VIR	24 LIB	24 SCO
28 LIB	26 SCO	26 SCO	26 CAP	26 AQU	26 ARI	26 TAU	27 CAN	28 VIR	28 LIB	26 SCO	26 SAG
30 SCO		28 SAG	29 AQU	28 PIS	29 TAU	28 GEM	29 LEO	30 LIB	30 SCO	29 SAG	28 CAP
		30 CAP		30 ARI		30 CAN	31 VIR				31 AQU

250

Moon Ephemeris: How to Find Your Moon Sign

1998

JAN	FEB	MAR	APR	MAY	JUN	JUL	AUG	SEP	OCT	NOV	DEC
2 PIS	2 TAU	2 TAU	2 CAN	2 LEO	3 LIB	3 SCO	2 SAG	3 AQU	2 PIS	1 ARI	2 GEM
4 ARI	4 GEM	4 GEM	4 LEO	4 VIR	5 SCO	5 SAG	4 CAP	5 PIS	4 ARI	3 TAU	4 CAN
6 TAU	7 CAN	6 CAN	7 VIR	7 LIB	8 SAG	8 CAP	6 AQU	7 ARI	6 TAU	5 GEM	6 LEO
8 GEM	9 LEO	8 LEO	9 LIB	9 SCO	10 CAP	10 AQU	8 PIS	9 TAU	8 GEM	7 CAN	9 VIR
10 CAN	11 VIR	11 VIR	12 SCO	12 SAG	13 AQU	12 PIS	11 ARI	11 GEM	10 CAN	9 LEO	11 LIB
13 LEO	14 LIB	13 LIB	14 SAG	14 CAP	15 PIS	14 ARI	13 TAU	13 CAN	13 LEO	11 VIR	14 SCO
15 VIR	16 SCO	16 SCO	17 CAP	16 AQU	17 ARI	16 TAU	15 GEM	15 LEO	15 VIR	14 LIB	16 SAG
18 LIB	19 SAG	18 SAG	19 AQU	19 PIS	19 TAU	18 GEM	17 CAN	18 VIR	17 LIB	16 SCO	19 CAP
20 SCO	21 CAP	21 CAP	21 PIS	21 ARI	21 GEM	21 CAN	19 LEO	20 LIB	20 SCO	19 SAG	21 AQU
23 SAG	23 AQU	23 AQU	23 ARI	23 TAU	23 CAN	23 LEO	21 VIR	23 SCO	23 SAG	21 CAP	23 PIS
25 CAP	25 PIS	25 PIS	25 TAU	25 GEM	25 LEO	25 VIR	24 LIB	25 SAG	25 CAP	24 AQU	25 ARI
27 AQU	27 ARI	27 ARI	27 GEM	27 CAN	28 VIR	28 LIB	26 SCO	28 CAP	27 AQU	26 PIS	28 TAU
29 PIS		29 TAU	29 CAN	29 LEO	30 LIB	30 SCO	29 SAG	30 AQU	30 PIS	28 ARI	30 GEM
31 ARI		31 GEM		31 VIR			31 CAP			30 TAU	

1999

JAN	FEB	MAR	APR	MAY	JUN	JUL	AUG	SEP	OCT	NOV	DEC
1 CAN	1 VIR	1 VIR	2 SCO	2 SAG	3 AQU	2 PIS	1 ARI	2 GEM	1 CAN	1 VIR	1 LIB
3 LEO	4 LIB	3 LIB	4 SAG	4 CAP	5 PIS	5 ARI	3 TAU	4 CAN	3 LEO	4 LIB	3 SCO
5 VIR	6 SCO	6 SCO	7 CAP	7 AQU	8 ARI	7 TAU	5 GEM	6 LEO	5 VIR	6 SCO	6 SAG
7 LIB	9 SAG	8 SAG	9 AQU	9 PIS	10 TAU	9 GEM	7 CAN	8 VIR	8 LIB	9 SAG	8 CAP
10 SCO	11 CAP	11 CAP	11 PIS	11 ARI	12 GEM	11 CAN	9 LEO	10 LIB	10 SCO	11 CAP	11 AQU
12 SAG	14 AQU	13 AQU	14 ARI	13 TAU	14 CAN	13 LEO	12 VIR	13 SCO	12 SAG	14 AQU	13 PIS
15 CAP	16 PIS	15 PIS	16 TAU	15 GEM	16 LEO	15 VIR	14 LIB	15 SAG	15 CAP	16 PIS	16 ARI
17 AQU	18 ARI	17 ARI	18 GEM	17 CAN	18 VIR	17 LIB	16 SCO	18 CAP	17 AQU	18 ARI	18 TAU
19 PIS	20 TAU	19 TAU	20 CAN	19 LEO	20 LIB	20 SCO	19 SAG	20 AQU	20 PIS	21 TAU	20 GEM
22 ARI	22 GEM	21 GEM	22 LEO	21 VIR	23 SCO	22 SAG	21 CAP	22 PIS	22 ARI	23 GEM	22 CAN
24 TAU	24 CAN	23 CAN	24 VIR	24 LIB	25 SAG	25 CAP	24 AQU	25 ARI	24 TAU	25 CAN	24 LEO
26 GEM	26 LEO	26 LEO	27 LIB	26 SCO	28 CAP	27 AQU	26 PIS	27 TAU	26 GEM	27 LEO	26 VIR
28 CAN		28 VIR	29 SCO	29 SAG	30 AQU	30 PIS	28 ARI	29 GEM	28 CAN	29 VIR	28 LIB
30 LEO		30 LIB		31 CAP			30 TAU		30 LEO		31 SCO

2000

JAN	FEB	MAR	APR	MAY	JUN	JUL	AUG	SEP	OCT	NOV	DEC
3 SAG	1 CAP	2 AQU	1 PIS	3 TAU	1 GEM	1 LEO	1 VIR	2 SCO	1 SAG	3 AQU	2 PIS
5 CAP	4 AQU	4 PIS	3 ARI	5 GEM	3 CAN	4 VIR	3 LIB	4 SAG	4 CAP	5 PIS	5 ARI
7 AQU	6 PIS	7 ARI	5 TAU	7 CAN	5 LEO	7 LIB	5 SCO	6 CAP	6 AQU	8 ARI	7 TAU
10 PIS	8 ARI	9 TAU	7 GEM	9 LEO	7 VIR	9 SCO	8 SAG	9 AQU	9 PIS	10 TAU	9 GEM
12 ARI	11 TAU	11 GEM	9 CAN	11 VIR	9 LIB	11 SAG	10 CAP	11 PIS	11 ARI	12 GEM	11 CAN
14 TAU	13 GEM	13 CAN	11 LEO	13 LIB	12 SCO	14 CAP	13 AQU	14 ARI	13 TAU	14 CAN	13 LEO
16 GEM	15 CAN	15 LEO	14 VIR	15 SCO	14 SAG	16 AQU	15 PIS	16 TAU	16 GEM	16 LEO	15 VIR
18 CAN	17 LEO	17 VIR	16 LIB	18 SAG	17 CAP	19 PIS	18 ARI	18 GEM	18 CAN	18 VIR	18 LIB
20 LEO	19 VIR	20 LIB	18 SCO	20 CAP	19 AQU	21 ARI	20 TAU	20 CAN	20 LEO	20 LIB	20 SCO
23 VIR	21 LIB	22 SCO	21 SAG	23 AQU	22 PIS	24 TAU	22 GEM	23 LEO	23 VIR	23 SCO	22 SAG
25 LIB	23 SCO	24 SAG	23 CAP	25 PIS	24 ARI	26 GEM	24 CAN	25 VIR	24 LIB	25 SAG	25 CAP
27 SCO	26 SAG	27 CAP	26 AQU	28 ARI	26 TAU	28 CAN	26 LEO	27 LIB	27 SCO	27 CAP	27 AQU
29 SAG	28 CAP	29 AQU	28 PIS	30 TAU	28 GEM	30 LEO	28 VIR	29 SCO	29 SAG	29 AQU	30 PIS
			30 ARI		30 CAN		30 LIB		31 CAP		

2001

JAN	FEB	MAR	APR	MAY	JUN	JUL	AUG	SEP	OCT	NOV	DEC
1 ARI	2 GEM	1 GEM	2 LEO	1 VIR	2 SCO	1 SAG	3 AQU	1 PIS	1 ARI	2 GEM	2 CAN
4 TAU	4 CAN	4 CAN	4 VIR	3 LIB	4 SAG	4 CAP	5 PIS	4 ARI	4 TAU	4 CAN	4 LEO
6 GEM	6 LEO	6 LEO	6 LIB	5 SCO	7 CAP	6 AQU	8 ARI	6 TAU	6 GEM	7 LEO	6 VIR
8 CAN	8 VIR	8 VIR	8 SCO	8 SAG	9 AQU	9 PIS	10 TAU	8 GEM	8 CAN	9 VIR	8 LIB
10 LEO	10 LIB	10 LIB	10 SAG	10 CAP	11 PIS	11 ARI	12 GEM	11 CAN	10 LEO	11 LIB	10 SCO
12 VIR	12 SCO	12 SCO	13 CAP	13 AQU	14 ARI	14 TAU	14 CAN	13 LEO	13 VIR	13 SCO	12 SAG
14 LIB	15 SAG	14 SAG	15 AQU	15 PIS	16 TAU	16 GEM	16 LEO	15 VIR	15 LIB	15 SAG	15 CAP
16 SCO	17 CAP	17 CAP	18 PIS	18 ARI	19 GEM	18 CAN	19 VIR	17 LIB	17 SCO	17 CAP	17 AQU
18 SAG	20 AQU	19 AQU	20 ARI	20 TAU	21 CAN	20 LEO	21 LIB	19 SCO	19 SAG	20 AQU	20 PIS
21 CAP	22 PIS	22 PIS	23 TAU	22 GEM	23 LEO	22 VIR	23 SCO	21 SAG	21 CAP	22 PIS	22 ARI
23 AQU	25 ARI	24 ARI	25 GEM	25 CAN	25 VIR	24 LIB	25 SAG	24 CAP	23 AQU	25 ARI	25 TAU
26 PIS	27 TAU	26 TAU	27 CAN	27 LEO	27 LIB	26 SCO	27 CAP	26 AQU	26 PIS	27 TAU	27 GEM
28 ARI		29 GEM	29 LEO	29 VIR	29 SCO	29 SAG	30 AQU	29 PIS	28 ARI	30 GEM	29 CAN
31 TAU		31 CAN		31 LIB		31 CAP			31 TAU		31 LEO

2002

JAN	FEB	MAR	APR	MAY	JUN	JUL	AUG	SEP	OCT	NOV	DEC
2 VIR	1 LIB	2 SCO	1 SAG	2 AQU	1 PIS	1 ARI	2 GEM	1 CAN	1 LEO	1 LIB	1 SCO
4 LIB	3 SCO	4 SAG	3 CAP	5 PIS	4 ARI	4 TAU	5 CAN	3 LEO	3 VIR	3 SCO	3 SAG
6 SCO	5 SAG	6 CAP	5 AQU	7 ARI	6 TAU	7 GEM	7 LEO	5 VIR	5 LIB	5 SAG	5 CAP
9 SAG	7 CAP	9 AQU	8 PIS	10 TAU	9 GEM	9 CAN	9 VIR	7 LIB	7 SCO	7 CAP	7 AQU
11 CAP	10 AQU	11 PIS	10 ARI	12 GEM	11 CAN	11 LEO	11 LIB	9 SCO	9 SAG	10 AQU	9 PIS
13 AQU	12 PIS	14 ARI	13 TAU	15 CAN	13 LEO	13 VIR	13 SCO	12 SAG	11 CAP	12 PIS	12 ARI
16 PIS	15 ARI	16 TAU	15 GEM	17 LEO	15 VIR	15 LIB	15 SAG	14 CAP	14 AQU	15 ARI	14 TAU
18 ARI	17 TAU	19 GEM	18 CAN	19 VIR	17 LIB	17 SCO	18 CAP	16 AQU	16 PIS	17 TAU	17 GEM
21 TAU	20 GEM	21 CAN	20 LEO	21 LIB	20 SCO	19 SAG	20 AQU	19 PIS	19 ARI	20 GEM	19 CAN
23 GEM	22 CAN	24 LEO	22 VIR	23 SCO	22 SAG	21 CAP	22 PIS	21 ARI	21 TAU	22 CAN	22 LEO
26 CAN	24 LEO	26 VIR	24 LIB	25 SAG	24 CAP	24 AQU	25 ARI	24 TAU	24 GEM	24 LEO	24 VIR
28 LEO	26 VIR	28 LIB	26 SCO	27 CAP	26 AQU	26 PIS	27 TAU	26 GEM	26 CAN	27 VIR	26 LIB
30 VIR	28 LIB	30 SCO	28 SAG	29 AQU	29 PIS	29 ARI	30 GEM	29 CAN	28 LEO	29 LIB	28 SCO
			30 CAP			31 TAU			30 VIR		30 SAG

251

Healing Mind, Body, Spirit

2003

JAN	FEB	MAR	APR	MAY	JUN	JUL	AUG	SEP	OCT	NOV	DEC
1 CAP	2 PIS	1 PIS	3 TAU	2 GEM	1 CAN	1 LEO	2 LIB	2 SAG	1 CAP	2 PIS	2 ARI
3 AQU	5 ARI	4 ARI	5 GEM	5 CAN	4 LEO	3 VIR	4 SCO	4 CAP	4 AQU	5 ARI	4 TAU
6 PIS	7 TAU	6 TAU	8 CAN	7 LEO	6 VIR	5 LIB	6 SAG	6 AQU	6 PIS	7 TAU	7 GEM
8 ARI	10 GEM	9 GEM	10 LEO	10 VIR	8 LIB	7 SCO	8 CAP	9 PIS	8 ARI	10 GEM	9 CAN
11 TAU	12 CAN	11 CAN	12 VIR	12 LIB	10 SCO	10 SAG	10 AQU	11 ARI	11 TAU	12 CAN	12 LEO
13 GYM	14 LEO	14 LEO	14 LIB	14 SCO	12 SAG	12 CAP	12 PIS	13 TAU	13 GEM	15 LEO	14 VIR
16 CAN	16 VIR	16 VIR	16 SCO	16 SAG	14 CAP	14 AQU	15 ARI	16 GEM	16 CAN	17 VIR	16 LIB
18 LEO	18 LIB	18 LIB	18 SAG	18 CAP	16 AQU	16 PIS	17 TAU	18 CAN	18 LEO	19 LIB	19 SCO
20 VIR	21 SCO	20 SCO	20 CAP	20 AQU	19 PIS	18 ARI	20 GEM	21 LEO	21 VIR	21 SCO	21 SAG
22 LIB	23 SAG	22 SAG	23 AQU	22 PIS	21 ARI	21 TAU	22 CAN	23 VIR	23 LIB	23 SAG	23 CAP
24 SCO	25 CAP	24 CAP	25 PIS	25 ARI	24 TAU	23 GEM	25 LEO	25 LIB	25 SCO	25 CAP	25 AQU
26 SAG	27 AQU	26 AQU	27 ARI	27 TAU	26 GEM	26 CAN	27 VIR	27 SCO	27 SAG	27 AQU	27 PIS
29 CAP		29 PIS	30 TAU	30 GEM	28 CAN	28 LEO	29 LIB	29 SAG	29 CAP	29 PIS	29 ARI
31 AQU		31 ARI				30 VIR	31 SCO		31 AQU		

2004

JAN	FEB	MAR	APR	MAY	JUN	JUL	AUG	SEP	OCT	NOV	DEC
1 TAU	2 CAN	3 LEO	1 VIR	1 LIB	2 SAG	1 CAP	1 PIS	2 TAU	2 GEM	1 CAN	1 LEO
3 CEM	4 LEO	5 VIR	4 LIB	3 SCO	4 CAP	3 AQU	4 ARI	5 GEM	5 CAN	3 LEO	3 VIR
6 CAN	7 VIR	7 LIB	6 SCO	5 SAG	6 AQU	5 PIS	6 TAU	7 CAN	7 LEO	6 VIR	6 LIB
8 LEO	9 LIB	9 SCO	9 SAG	7 CAP	8 PIS	7 ARI	8 GEM	10 LEO	10 VIR	8 LIB	8 SCO
10 VIR	11 SCO	12 SAG	11 CAP	9 AQU	10 ARI	10 TAU	11 CAN	12 VIR	12 LIB	10 SCO	10 SAG
13 LIB	13 SAG	14 CAP	12 AQU	11 PIS	12 TAU	12 GEM	13 LEO	14 LIB	14 SCO	13 SAG	12 CAP
15 SCO	15 CAP	16 AQU	14 PIS	14 ARI	15 GEM	15 CAN	16 VIR	17 SCO	16 SAG	15 CAP	14 AQU
17 SAG	17 AQU	18 PIS	16 ARI	16 TAU	17 CAN	17 LEO	18 LIB	19 SAG	18 CAP	17 AQU	16 PIS
19 CAP	20 PIS	20 ARI	19 TAU	19 GEM	20 LEO	20 VIR	20 SCO	21 CAP	20 AQU	19 PIS	18 ARI
21 AQU	22 ARI	23 TAU	21 GEM	21 CAN	22 VIR	22 LIB	23 SAG	23 AQU	23 PIS	21 ARI	21 TAU
23 PIS	24 TAU	25 GEM	24 CAN	24 LEO	25 LIB	24 SCO	25 CAP	25 PIS	25 ARI	23 TAU	23 GEM
25 ARI	27 GEM	28 CAN	26 LEO	26 VIR	27 SCO	26 SAG	27 AQU	27 ARI	27 TAU	26 GEM	25 CAN
28 TAU	29 CAN	30 LEO	29 VIR	28 LIB	29 SAG	28 CAP	29 PIS	30 TAU	29 GEM	28 CAN	28 LEO
30 GEM				31 SCO		30 AQU	31 ARI				31 VIR

2005

JAN	FEB	MAR	APR	MAY	JUN	JUL	AUG	SEP	OCT	NOV	DEC
2 LIB	1 SCO	2 SAG	3 AQU	2 PIS	3 TAU	2 GEM	1 CAN	2 VIR	2 LIB	1 SCO	2 CAP
4 SCO	3 SAG	4 CAP	5 PIS	4 ARI	5 GEM	5 CAN	3 LEO	5 LIB	4 SCO	3 SAG	4 AQU
6 SAG	5 CAP	6 AQU	7 ARI	6 TAU	7 CAN	7 LEO	6 VIR	7 SCO	7 SAG	5 CAP	7 PIS
8 CAP	7 AQU	8 PIS	9 TAU	9 GEM	10 LEO	10 VIR	8 LIB	9 SAG	9 CAP	7 AQU	9 ARI
10 AQU	9 PIS	10 ARI	11 GEM	11 CAN	12 VIR	12 LIB	11 SCO	12 CAP	11 AQU	9 PIS	11 TAU
12 PIS	11 ARI	13 TAU	14 CAN	14 LEO	15 LIB	15 SCO	13 SAG	14 AQU	13 PIS	11 ARI	13 GEM
15 ARI	13 TAU	15 GEM	16 LEO	16 VIR	17 SCO	17 SAG	15 CAP	15 AQU	15 ARI	14 TAU	15 CAN
17 TAU	16 GEM	17 CAN	19 VIR	18 LIB	19 SAG	19 CAP	17 AQU	18 ARI	17 TAU	16 GEM	18 LEO
19 GEM	18 CAN	20 LEO	21 LIB	21 SCO	21 CAP	21 AQU	19 PIS	20 TAU	19 GEM	18 CAN	20 VIR
22 CAN	21 LEO	22 VIR	23 SCO	23 SAG	23 AQU	23 PIS	21 ARI	22 GEM	21 CAN	21 LEO	23 LIB
24 LEO	23 VIR	25 LIB	26 SAG	25 CAP	25 PIS	25 ARI	23 TAU	24 CAN	24 LEO	23 VIR	25 SCO
27 VIR	25 LIB	27 SCO	28 CAP	27 AQU	27 ARI	27 TAU	26 GEM	27 LEO	27 VIR	26 LIB	28 SAG
29 LIB	28 SCO	29 SAG	30 AQU	29 PIS	30 TAU	29 GEM	28 CAN	29 VIR	29 LIB	28 SCO	30 CAP
		31 CAP		31 ARI			31 LEO			30 SAG	

2006

JAN	FEB	MAR	APR	MAY	JUN	JUL	AUG	SEP	OCT	NOV	DEC
1 AQU	1 ARI	1 ARI	1 GEM	1 CAN	2 VIR	2 LIB	1 SCO	2 CAP	1 AQU	2 ARI	1 TAU
3 PIS	3 TAU	3 TAU	4 CAN	3 LEO	5 LIB	5 SCO	3 SAG	4 AQU	4 PIS	4 TAU	3 GEM
5 ARI	6 GEM	5 GEM	6 LEO	6 VIR	7 SCO	7 SAG	6 CAP	6 PIS	6 ARI	6 GEM	6 CAN
7 TAU	8 CAN	7 CAN	9 VIR	8 LIB	10 SAG	9 CAP	8 AQU	8 ARI	8 TAU	8 CAN	8 LEO
9 GEM	10 LEO	10 LEO	11 LIB	11 SCO	12 CAP	11 AQU	10 PIS	10 TAU	10 GEM	10 LEO	10 VIR
12 CAN	13 VIR	12 VIR	14 SCO	13 SAG	14 AQU	13 PIS	12 ARI	12 GEM	12 CAN	13 VIR	13 LIB
14 LEO	16 LIB	15 LIB	16 SAG	15 CAP	15 PIS	16 ARI	14 TAU	14 CAN	14 LEO	15 LIB	15 SCO
17 VIR	18 SCO	17 SCO	18 CAP	18 AQU	18 ARI	17 TAU	16 GEM	17 LEO	17 VIR	18 SCO	18 SAG
19 LIB	20 SAG	20 SAG	20 AQU	20 PIS	20 TAU	19 GEM	18 CAN	19 VIR	19 LIB	20 SAG	20 CAP
22 SCO	23 CAP	22 CAP	22 PIS	22 ARI	22 GEM	22 CAN	21 LEO	22 LIB	22 SCO	23 CAP	22 AQU
24 SAG	25 AQU	24 AQU	24 ARI	24 TAU	25 CAN	25 LEO	23 VIR	24 SCO	24 SAG	25 AQU	24 PIS
26 CAP	27 PIS	26 PIS	27 TAU	26 GEM	27 LEO	27 VIR	26 LIB	27 SAG	26 CAP	27 PIS	27 ARI
28 AQU		28 ARI	29 GEM	28 CAN	29 VIR	29 LIB	28 SCO	29 CAP	29 AQU	29 ARI	29 TAU
30 PIS		30 TAU		31 LEO			31 SAG		31 PIS		31 GEM

2007

JAN	FEB	MAR	APR	MAY	JUN	JUL	AUG	SEP	OCT	NOV	DEC
2 CAN	1 LEO	2 VIR	1 LIB	1 SCO	2 CAP	2 AQU	2 ARI	1 TAU	2 CAN	3 VIR	3 LIB
4 LEO	3 VIR	5 LIB	3 SCO	3 SAG	4 AQU	4 PIS	4 TAU	3 GEM	4 LEO	5 LIB	5 SCO
7 VIR	5 LIB	7 SCO	6 SAG	6 CAP	6 PIS	6 CEM	6 GEM	5 CAN	7 VIR	8 SCO	8 SAG
9 LIB	8 SCO	10 SAG	8 CAP	8 AQU	9 ARI	8 TAU	9 CAN	7 LEO	9 LIB	10 SAG	10 CAP
12 SCO	10 SAG	12 CAP	11 AQU	10 PIS	11 TAU	10 GEM	11 LEO	10 VIR	12 SCO	13 CAP	13 AQU
14 SAG	13 CAP	14 AQU	13 PIS	12 ARI	13 GEM	12 CAN	13 VIR	12 LIB	14 SAG	15 AQU	15 PIS
16 CAP	15 AQU	17 PIS	15 ARI	14 TAU	15 CAN	14 LEO	15 LIB	15 SCO	17 CAP	18 PIS	17 ARI
19 AQU	17 PIS	19 ARI	17 TAU	16 GEM	17 LEO	17 VIR	18 SCO	17 SAG	19 AQU	20 ARI	19 TAU
21 PIS	19 ARI	21 TAU	19 GEM	19 CAN	19 VIR	19 LIB	20 SAG	20 CAP	21 PIS	22 TAU	21 GEM
23 ARI	21 TAU	23 GEM	21 CAN	21 LEO	22 LIB	22 SCO	23 CAP	22 AQU	23 ARI	24 GEM	23 CAN
25 TAU	23 GEM	25 CAN	23 LEO	23 VIR	24 SCO	24 SAG	25 AQU	24 PIS	25 TAU	26 CAN	25 LEO
27 GEM	25 CAN	27 LEO	26 VIR	25 LIB	27 SAG	27 CAP	27 PIS	26 ARI	27 GEM	28 LEO	27 VIR
29 CAN	28 LEO	29 VIR	28 LIB	28 SCO	29 CAP	29 AQU	29 ARI	28 TAU	29 CAN	30 VIR	30 LIB
				31 SAG		31 PIS		30 GEM	31 LEO		

252

Moon Ephemeris: How to Find Your Moon Sign

2008

JAN	FEB	MAR	APR	MAY	JUN	JUL	AUG	SEP	OCT	NOV	DEC
1 SCO	3 CAP	1 CAP	2 PIS	2 ARI	2 GEM	2 CAN	2 VIR	1 LIB	3 SAG	2 CAP	2 AQU
4 SAG	5 AQU	3 AQU	4 ARI	4 TAU	4 CAN	4 LEO	4 LIB	3 SCO	5 CAP	4 AQU	4 PIS
6 CAP	7 PIS	6 PIS	6 TAU	6 GEM	6 LEO	6 VIR	7 SCO	6 SAG	8 AQU	7 PIS	6 ARI
9 AQU	10 ARI	8 ARI	8 GEM	8 CAN	8 VIR	8 LIB	9 SAG	8 CAP	10 PIS	9 ARI	9 TAU
11 PIS	12 TAU	10 TAU	10 CAN	10 LEO	10 LIB	10 SCO	12 CAP	11 AQU	13 ARI	11 TAU	11 GEM
13 ARI	14 GEM	12 GEM	13 LEO	12 VIR	13 SCO	13 SAG	14 AQU	13 PIS	15 TAU	13 GEM	13 CAN
15 TAU	16 CAN	14 CAN	15 VIR	14 LIB	16 SAG	15 CAP	17 PIS	15 ARI	17 GEM	15 CAN	15 LEO
18 GEM	18 LEO	16 LEO	17 LIB	17 SCO	18 CAP	18 AQU	19 ARI	17 TAU	19 CAN	17 LEO	17 VIR
20 CAN	20 VIR	19 VIR	20 SCO	19 SAG	21 AQU	20 PIS	21 TAU	19 GEM	21 LEO	19 VIR	19 LIB
22 LEO	23 LIB	21 LIB	22 SAG	22 CAP	23 PIS	23 GEM	23 CAN	22 CAN	23 VIR	22 LIB	21 SCO
24 VIR	25 SCO	23 SCO	25 CAP	24 AQU	25 ARI	25 TAU	25 CAN	24 LEO	25 LIB	24 SCO	24 SAG
26 LIB	23 SAG	26 SAG	27 AQU	27 PIS	28 TAU	27 GEM	27 LEO	26 VIR	28 SCO	27 SAG	26 CAP
29 SCO		28 CAP	30 PIS	29 ARI	30 GEM	29 CAN	30 VIR	28 LIB	30 SAG	29 CAP	29 AQU
31 SAG		31 AQU		31 TAU		31 LEO		30 SCO			31 PIS

2009

JAN	FEB	MAR	APR	MAY	JUN	JUL	AUG	SEP	OCT	NOV	DEC
3 ARI	1 TAU	3 GEM	1 CAN	2 VIR	1 LIB	3 SAG	2 CAP	3 PIS	3 ARI	1 TAU	1 GEM
5 TAU	3 GEM	5 CAN	3 LEO	5 LIB	3 SCO	5 CAP	4 AQU	5 ARI	5 TAU	4 GEM	3 CAN
7 GEM	5 CAN	7 LEO	5 VIR	7 SCO	6 SAG	8 AQU	7 PIS	8 TAU	7 GEM	6 CAN	5 LEO
9 CAN	7 LEO	9 VIR	7 LIB	9 SAG	8 CAP	10 PIS	9 ARI	10 GEM	9 CAN	8 LEO	7 VIR
11 LEO	10 VIR	11 LIB	10 SCO	12 CAP	11 AQU	13 ARI	11 TAU	12 CAN	12 LEO	10 VIR	9 LIB
13 VIR	12 LIB	13 SCO	12 SAG	14 AQU	13 PIS	15 TAU	14 GEM	14 LEO	14 VIR	12 LIB	11 SCO
15 LIB	14 SCO	16 SAG	15 CAP	17 PIS	16 ARI	17 GEM	16 CAN	16 VIR	16 LIB	14 SCO	14 SAG
18 SCO	16 SAG	18 CAP	17 AQU	19 ARI	18 TAU	19 CAN	18 LEO	18 LIB	18 SCO	17 SAG	16 CAP
20 SAG	19 CAP	21 AQU	20 PIS	21 TAU	20 GEM	21 LEO	20 VIR	20 SCO	20 SAG	19 CAP	19 AQU
23 CAP	21 AQU	23 PIS	22 ARI	24 GEM	22 CAN	23 VIR	22 LIB	23 SAG	23 CAP	21 AQU	21 PIS
25 AQU	24 PIS	26 ARI	24 TAU	26 CAN	24 LEO	25 LIB	25 SCO	25 CAP	25 AQU	24 PIS	24 ARI
28 PIS	26 ARI	28 TAU	26 GEM	28 LEO	26 VIR	28 SCO	26 SAG	28 AQU	28 PIS	26 ARI	26 TAU
30 ARI	28 TAU	30 GEM	28 CAN	30 VIR	28 LIB	30 SAG	29 CAP	30 PIS	30 ARI	29 TAU	28 GEM
			30 LEO		30 SCO		31 AQU				30 CAN

2010

JAN	FEB	MAR	APR	MAY	JUN	JUL	AUG	SEP	OCT	NOV	DEC
1 LEO	2 LIB	1 LIB	2 SAG	2 CAP	1 AQU	3 ARI	2 TAU	3 CAN	2 LEO	3 LIB	2 SCO
3 VIR	4 SCO	3 SCO	4 CAP	4 AQU	3 PIS	5 TAU	4 GEM	5 LEO	4 VIR	5 SCO	4 SAG
6 LIB	6 SAG	6 SAG	7 AQU	7 PIS	6 ARI	8 GEM	6 CAN	7 VIR	6 LIB	7 SAG	6 CAP
8 SCO	9 CAP	8 CAP	9 PIS	9 ARI	8 TAU	10 CAN	8 LEO	9 LIB	8 SCO	9 CAP	9 AQU
10 SAG	11 AQU	11 AQU	12 ARI	12 TAU	10 GEM	12 LEO	10 VIR	11 SCO	10 SAG	11 AQU	11 PIS
13 CAP	14 PIS	13 PIS	14 TAU	14 GEM	12 CAN	14 VIR	12 LIB	13 SAG	12 CAP	14 PIS	14 ARI
15 AQU	16 ARI	16 ARI	17 GEM	16 CAN	14 LEO	16 LIB	14 SCO	15 CAP	15 AQU	16 ARI	16 TAU
18 PIS	19 TAU	18 TAU	19 CAN	18 LEO	17 VIR	18 SCO	17 SAG	18 AQU	17 PIS	19 TAU	18 GEM
20 ARI	21 GEM	20 GEM	21 LEO	20 VIR	19 LIB	20 SAG	19 CAP	20 PIS	20 ARI	21 GEM	21 CAN
22 TAU	23 CAN	23 CAN	23 VIR	22 LIB	21 SCO	23 CAP	21 AQU	23 ARI	22 TAU	23 CAN	23 LEO
25 GEM	25 LEO	25 LEO	25 LIB	25 SCO	23 SAG	25 AQU	24 PIS	25 TAU	25 GEM	26 LEO	25 VIR
27 CAN	27 VIR	27 VIR	27 SCO	27 SAG	25 CAP	28 PIS	26 ARI	28 GEM	27 CAN	23 VIR	27 LIB
29 LEO		29 LIB	29 SAG	29 CAP	28 AQU	30 ARI	29 TAU	30 CAN	29 LEO	30 LIB	29 SCO
31 VIR		31 SCO			30 PIS		31 GEM		31 VIR		31 SAG

Astrological and Counseling Services

∽ To Contact the Author

To contact the author regarding personal appearances, or group seminars, write to:

M. J. Abadie c/o Hazelwood Productions
P.O. Box 247
Lenox Hill Station
New York, NY 10021

Please give particulars in your letter about your wishes.

∽ Astrological Services

We offer a range of computerized astrological services via mail. These include a Simple Natal Chart, Personal Profiles (a detailed analysis of your chart), the Relationship Profile (a compatibility analysis between two people), A Child's Profile, and outer-planet transit lists with individual interpretations, as well as personal, non-computer astrological readings by telephone.

To receive a free descriptive brochure, please send a stamped, self-addressed envelope to the address below. Canadian and other non-U.S. correspondents can send $1.00 in lieu of SASE to:

Hazelwood Productions
P.O. Box 247
Lenox Hill Station
New York, NY 10021

Also by M. J. Abadie

Your Psychic Potential

An outstanding guide for developing the psychic talent that lies dormant in all of us, with practical steps that really work. The extraordinary power of psychics and psychic ability is a part of mainstream American culture. Yet most people do not realize they already possess the capacity to anticipate and guide major aspects of their lives. *Your Psychic Potential* shows how to gain access to your hidden skills of intuition, your subconscious, and your dreams, to uncover the secrets of your past and future. Recognizing and developing these gifts can help people improve relationships, solve financial problems, find the right job, increase self-confidence, and attract a lifelong partner. This exciting book allows you to explore and master your own psychic power.

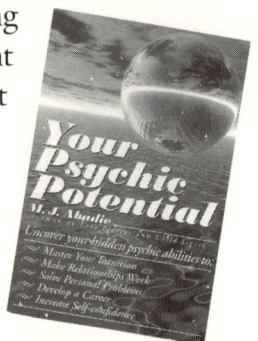

6" x 9", 320 pages, $10.95, trade paperback

Available wherever books are sold

If you cannot find these titles at your favorite retail outlet, you may order them directly from the publisher. BY PHONE: Call 1-800-872-5627 (in Massachusetts 617-767-8100). We accept Visa, Mastercard, and American Express. $4.50 will be added to your total order for shipping and handling. BY MAIL: Write out the full titles of the books you'd like to order and send payment, including $4.50 for shipping and handling, to: Adams Media Corporation, 260 Center Street, Holbrook, MA 02343. 30-day money-back guarantee.